The Case for
American Medicine

A REALISTIC LOOK AT
OUR HEALTH CARE SYSTEM

OTHER BOOKS BY HARRY SCHWARTZ

Seasonal Migratory Agricultural Labor in the United States

Eastern Europe in the Soviet Shadow

Prague's 200 Days, The Struggle for Democracy in Czechoslovakia

Tsars, Mandarins and Commissars: A History of Chinese-Russian Relations

An Introduction to the Soviet Economy

China

The Soviet Economy Since Stalin

The Many Faces of Communism (editor)

The Red Phoenix: Russia Since World War II

Russia's Soviet Economy

Soviet Union: Communist Economic Power

Russia's Postwar Economy

Russia Enters the 1960's (editor)

The Case for American Medicine

A REALISTIC LOOK AT
OUR HEALTH CARE SYSTEM

by Harry Schwartz

DAVID McKAY COMPANY, INC.   New York

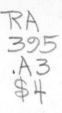

THE CASE FOR AMERICAN MEDICINE
A Realistic Look at Our Health Care System

FIFTH PRINTING, OCTOBER 1973

LIBRARY OF CONGRESS CATALOG CARD NUMBER: 72-90173

MANUFACTURED IN THE UNITED STATES OF AMERICA

For Stephanie, Bonnie, and David

CONTENTS

INTRODUCTION

In his *Devil's Dictionary*, Ambrose Bierce defined a physician as "one upon whom we set our hopes when ill and our dogs when well." The definition is still apt today, especially if we apply it to the total American medical system and not merely to physicians. American medicine is now at the height of its capability, providing more—and more effective—help to a larger number of our people than ever before. At almost every point along the frontiers of the fight against death and disability American physicians and medical researchers are the world leaders. They are setting new standards of excellence in such diverse fields as heart and kidney transplants, knee and hip replacements, treatment of leukemia and hypertension, the prevention of RH incompatibility and the application of new weapons against hyaline membrane disease in newborn babies. Yet never before has so ferocious an attack upon American medicine been mounted as in recent years, an attack that too often leaves the highroad of reasoned criticism and descends to emotionalism and misrepresentation.

This book is an attempt to tell the other side of the

story, to help turn the national discussion of medical-care delivery into more of a debate and less of a dreary repetition of inaccurate clichés. I have attempted in this volume to confront the most frequent criticisms of American medicine and to examine the relevant evidence available for reaching judgments on these criticisms. I have also probed here into the favorite "solutions" offered by critics, and have tried to examine these "solutions" with better information than their advocates seem usually to possess. The reader will see that I am under no illusion American medicine is perfect or beyond improving. I am also well aware that particular institutions and individuals in the American medical system may perform below par and deserve severe criticism. But to recognize that American medicine is composed of fallible human beings and has inadequacies in need of remedy is a far cry from the critics' stereotyped claim that we are in a "health care crisis" of such magnitude and gravity that only the most radical surgery will set matters aright.

Two main techniques are employed by the most extreme critics of American medicine. One is to collect a number of case histories about individuals who have allegedly been mistreated, bankrupted, or victimized by American medicine, and then to present this collection of unrepresentative horror stories as the essential truth about this nation's medical system. Unfortunately, this kind of unfair and one-sided approach dominates much of the contemporary discussion of this field by politicians and journalists.

An alternative technique is to set up a utopian picture of what medical care might be like in some perfect world dreamed up by a writer of science fiction, and then to list the ways in which the reality of American medicine differs from it. By that technique, of course, every American institution would be found wanting, since none meets utopian standards. One variant of this device is to select some foreign medical system, British, Swedish, or Russian, for instance, about which it may be assumed most Americans know little or nothing. Then the critic points out the areas in which he believes this foreign medical system is better than the American, and generalizes about the overall superiority he claims for the foreign medical system. Every nation's medical system has faults; in every country there are frequent complaints about medical shortcomings, but this is never mentioned. Sometimes, of course, the critic is self-deceived, a victim of his own ignorance. A well-known journalist, for example, created a stir some time ago by publishing a comparison of American and British health statistics which showed the apparent superiority of the British medical system. But further investigation showed that the British and American data used were not comparable, and that therefore the published comparison was meaningless.

In writing this book I have had generous help from many people. My chief debt is to my wife, Ruth B. Schwartz, who has aided me in every phase of the research and thought that have gone into this volume. I have benefited greatly from the suggestions made by friends who have read the manuscript and criticized it, notably Helen Avnet and Miriam Ostow, both medical economists, and Philip Aisen, M.D., and David V. Habif, M.D., among others. In addition, Bernard Albert, M.D., read and commented helpfully on the chapter on Health Maintenance Organizations. But I did not accept all of the suggestions offered, so the full blame for any errors is mine alone.

Dorothy P. Rice of the Department of Health, Education and Welfare supplied much useful material, as did various representatives of the National Center for Health Statistics, the American Hospital Association, the American Medical Association, the Blue Cross and Blue Shield organizations, and the California Medical Association. Many members of the Kaiser-Permanente organization were generous in sharing their knowledge, and I am particularly grateful for the courtesies shown me by Sidney Garfield, M.D., Arthur Weissman, Avram Yedidia, and John M. Mott, M.D. I also received much valuable information from personnel connected with several medical foundations, particularly one in Sacramento, California, and with various neighborhood health centers. And I cannot fail to mention the private physicians who have treated me and my family so effectively in many medical crises over the past quarter of a century, demonstrating repeatedly their excellence as compassionate and skilled healers.

My thanks are due also to the Commonwealth Fund and the Brookings Institution for permission to reproduce copyright material from books they have published.

The opinions in this book are strictly my own, and do not necessarily reflect those of the persons named nor of my employers, *The New York Times* and the State University of New York.

Harry Schwartz
September 1972

The Case for American Medicine

A REALISTIC LOOK AT
OUR HEALTH CARE SYSTEM

CHAPTER I

THE AMERICAN
MEDICAL SYSTEM

The following letter appeared in the August 11, 1972 issue of *Life* magazine:

We were a young couple, new to a strange town, when my wife became ill. I located the only doctor in the area who had Wednesday office hours. He saw us early that evening, diagnosed the problem, called in a specialist and arranged to admit my wife to a hospital. At midnight the specialist, who we later learned was the best in the area, and the general practitioner, whom we had never met before, operated on my wife. Without the operation, she would not have lived until morning.

The letter appeared in connection with the magazine's report on the response 41,000 *Life* readers had made to a poll on how they felt about the medical care they and their families receive. It is not unlikely that *Life*'s editors expected the results of their poll might be overwhelmingly against the American medical system. Not too long before the poll, *Life* had printed a full-page editorial denouncing "Our Sick Medical System." But when its readers' opinions were in, *Life* reported the answers reflected "a surprising degree of satisfaction with the treatment received" and that the letter quoted above expresses "a sense of gratitude and trust that many people still have for doctors." Of the *Life* readers who responded, 68 percent rated their medical treatment good to excellent and 70 percent said their doctor cared about them personally. *Life* noted that "only one reader in 15 considers his medical care 'poor,' and just one in 20 thinks his doctor is 'indifferent.' "

Life was careful to point out that the 41,000 readers responding to its poll were not "a scientifically calculated cross section of the nation" and that the respondents were above average in education. But other polls have shown similar results. They have also indicated that there is a vast reservoir of trust and confidence in Amercan medicine among a majority of this nation's people.

But anybody who has followed the coverage of American medicine in the media these past several years knows that a very different tone has predominated. The emphasis has been along the lines of *Life*'s editorial titled "Our Sick Medical System," with both commentary and reporting emphasizing alleged defects and demanding radical change. It has been an unfair and often inaccurate chorus of condemnation prompted more by ideological preconceptions and inadequate understanding than by the reality. American medicine is probably, on the whole and with exceptions in particular areas, the best in the world. But one who took seriously the massive propaganda offensive of recent years could easily believe that American medicine was in terrible shape, and was failing its obligations to the American people in almost every respect. The influence of these preconceptions on much journalistic discussion of American medicine may be illustrated by the following curious recent example:

On October 23, 1971, the *Washington Post*'s correspon-

dent in Moscow, Robert G. Kaiser, reported some of his
first impressions and experiences in the Soviet capital. He
had found "the mundane reality of the Soviet Union . . .
startling," he admitted, and full of surprises. As one example he told of a cab ride during which the "lady taxi
driver startled me by blurting out—after I said I was an
American—'In your country, everything is better, right?'
After several seconds of flustered silence I felt relieved to
be able to say, 'No, ordinary people in my country have
worse medical care than you do.' "

How did the correspondent—newly arrived and just getting his bearings—know that ordinary people in the United
States "have worse medical care" than their Soviet counter-
parts? He gave no evidence and seemed to feel none was
necessary. Mr. Kaiser had apparently never read Alexander
Solzhenitsyn's great novel *Cancer Ward,* in which a character obviously speaking for the Nobel laureate Soviet author
sneers at the socialized Soviet medical system, asking, "Is
this in fact such a great achievement? What does 'free'
mean? The doctors don't work for nothing, you know. It
only means that they're paid out of the national budget and
the budget is supported by patients. It isn't free treatment,
it's depersonalized treatment. . . . You would be ready to
pay goodness knows how much for a decent reception at
the doctor's, but there's no one to go [to] to get it. They all
have their schedules and their quotas, and so it's 'Next patient, please.' " Mr. Kaiser had obviously also not read Solzhenitsyn's moving story, "The Right Hand," an appalling
tale of the callousness shown toward a terminal cancer victim seeking admission to a Soviet hospital.

In June 1972 the distinguished Soviet physicist and
fighter for Soviet civil liberties, Academician Andrei D.
Sakharov, made available to foreign correspondents in

Moscow a memorandum he had written regarding conditions in his country. Part of this memorandum gave Academician Sakharov's judgment of Soviet education and medical care for ordinary citizens and sounded almost as though this distinguished scientist had been reading Mr. Kaiser's pronouncements on Soviet health care. Academician Sakharov wrote: "The deplorable condition of popular education and health care is carefully hidden from foreign eyes, but for all those who wish to see, it cannot be a secret. The free system of health care and education is no more than an economic illusion in a society where all surplus value is expropriated and distributed by the government. The hierarchical class structure of our society with its system of privileges has been especially perniciously reflected in health care and education. The condition of education and health care for the people—this is the destitution of the open admission hospitals, the poverty and oppression of the teacher." Academician Sakharov's prescription for improving the Soviet medical system was phrased in these terms: "Concerning reform of the system of health care we must: expand the network of polyclinics and hospitals requiring payment of fees; increase the role of physicians, registered nurses, and practical nurses in private practice; increase the wages of medical workers at all levels . . ."

The *Washington Post*'s correspondent is hardly unique in denigrating American medicine. A host of journalists and politicians have been seeking to convince the American people in recent years that they suffer from what is variously called a "health care crisis" or "health crisis." *Fortune* magazine, for example, has called the nation's physicians "an army of pushcart vendors in an age of supermarkets," adding that "American medicine, the pride of the nation for many years, stands now on the brink of chaos." But as this is written, almost three years later, that "brink" has not been crossed. In a widely viewed television special, the Columbia Broadcasting System paraded a group of horror stories about American medicine before its audience, warning viewers, "Don't Get Sick in America." Unfortunately, CBS failed to inform its audience where in the world it is a good idea to get sick, to become a victim, say, of cancer, multiple sclerosis, or schizophrenia. *Look* magazine, in one of its last issues, blazoned across its front cover the words, "Why You Can't Get a Doctor," though its editors must have known that millions of Americans see doctors every week. Many more examples of rhetorical overkill could be cited, all parts of a major effort to convince Americans that medical care in this country is second-rate and sinfully expensive. It has all been reminiscent of the simplistic anti-Soviet and anti-Chinese propaganda of the worst Cold War days.

The other side of this vast brainwashing effort has been the equally simplistic effort to convince Americans that there are easy solutions to the supposed "medical mess." Nothing less than a total revolution is required, the reformers have insisted. Detailed prescriptions have varied from critic to critic but the essentials have been similar. The faults of American medicine, it has been said, result from the fact that it is a "cottage industry" and a "nonsystem" dominated by "solo practitioners" working on a "fee for service" basis.

American medicine has to be made a "system," we have been told repeatedly. The direct financial relationship between doctor and patient must be abolished and all medical care made "free" through national health insurance or its equivalent. "Solo practitioners," allegedly growing rich in their neighborhood offices, must be driven from their golden ghettoes and compelled to accept collectivization, to join prepaid group practices. After this, it is claimed, the way will finally be open to alleviate America's ills, cut the death rate, and make free, first-class medical care available equally to all Americans.

The most enthusiastic utopians propounding these doctrines conjure up happy visions of the day when the poorest black Alabama sharecropper will have available the same standard of medical care as, say, Senator Edward M. Kennedy. But no such equality exists anywhere in the world. Does anyone seriously believe, for example, that Mao Tsetung or Chou En-lai has no better medical care available than any Chinese peasant tending rice fields? When James Reston of *The New York Times* was struck down by appendicitis in Peking in 1971 the Chinese government saw to it that he had eleven specialists in attendance for his diagnosis, surgery, and postoperative treatment. That would be extraordinary care in any country, let alone an underdeveloped nation such as China. In the Soviet Union the existence of special closed medical facilities for the Kremlin leaders and for other important Soviet figures is well known. Some years ago when the great Soviet physicist, Lev Landau, was badly injured in an accident literally dozens of Soviet physicians were assigned to his care, while some outstanding foreign specialists were brought to the Soviet Union to aid in his treatment. When the then Soviet Premier, Nikita S. Khrushchev, was in the United States in 1959 he had his own personal physician with him. As Solzhenitsyn has shown us, this abundance of medical care for the elite is far from typical of Soviet medicine for the masses.

Those who denounce the American medical system because it does not meet the criteria of their utopian blueprint forget the limitations of even the best medical system and of the best care for even the most powerful or richest individual. All human beings die eventually. No medical system, regardless of how it is organized, can save persons killed on impact in airplane crashes, like Walter Reuther, or those who are victims of bullets shot into vital organs, like John and Robert Kennedy, or those afflicted with incurable cancer, like John Foster Dulles, or those who kill themselves swiftly with a drug overdose, like so tragically many young people.

This book will demonstrate that a "health care crisis" or a "health crisis," in the terms the propagandists usually present the matter, does not exist. It will also focus attention on the many positive qualities of American medicine that normally escape the attention of the critics. Every American who suffers from advanced cancer or other life-threatening disease is, of course, the victim of a major personal crisis. The same thing is true, however, of every other person in the world who has advanced cancer or some similar terrible ailment. No medical system provides immortality, and all human beings eventually die.

The positive evaluation of most of American medicine given here is not intended to deny that there are serious problems and deficiencies or that further improvement is necessary. But rational judgment requires that those who want to improve matters be aware that American medicine has strengths as well as weaknesses. Any proposal for radical change must be examined with an eye to the possible damage it can do to the many areas of excellence in American medical care as well as with an eye to possible gains in areas of deficiency. In any case, whatever organizational reforms are proposed or implemented, most medical care in this country for the next generation will be delivered primarily by today's physicians, who are so often slandered by those who dream of a medical Utopia. Regardless of how attractive its theoretical blueprint may seem, no new American medical system can work well if it is imposed upon the nation's physicians, dentists and other health service personnel against their will and without consideration for their ideas and legitimate interests.

To date the campaign of denigration directed against American medicine has not succeeded to the extent the propagandists had hoped. The gap between the reality most Americans observe in their contacts with the medical system and the monstrous scarecrow depicted in the propaganda has been too wide. The great popularity of a television program like Marcus Welby, M.D.—which conveys a warm, positive image of physicians—would not be possible if most Americans saw their doctors as the grim, cold, and hostile figures the most impassioned critics depict. In late 1971 the backers of the Kennedy national health insurance bill came close to throwing in the towel because, as the *New York Times* reported on December 19, 1971, the American "public has not given the massive support to the proposed program" that its sponsors had anticipated. This failure of the American people to respond is particularly impressive when one remembers the widespread campaign Senator Kennedy, the union movement, some businessmen, and some influential journalists have mounted to whip up a public demand for radical change.

The basic reason for the disappointment of the Kennedy forces was the fact that the United States has a very large, well-equipped, and generally high quality medical system. Most Americans have access to this system and millions use it every week. The magnitude of the nation's medical organization is indicated by two statistics: In the early 1970s the United States was spending in excess of $70 billion annually for health care and related activities which employed a huge army of more than 4 million health workers.

The human resources available in the United States to meet its health care needs can be indicated most simply by listing the numbers in some of the key categories involved as listed in the U.S. Government publication *Health Resources Statistics:*

Physicians	323,000
Medical research scientists	51,200
Dentists	102,900
Dentists' aides	140,000
Registered nurses	723,000
Practical nurses	400,000
Nurses' aides, orderlies, etc.	850,000
Pharmacists and pharmacists' assistants	139,300
Clinical laboratory personnel	140,000
Optometry and optical services	35,000
X-ray technicians	75,000–100,000
Social workers	29,800
Physical therapists	24,000
Podiatrists	7,000
Speech pathologists and audiologists	19,000

These data apply to the year 1970. In 1972, there were probably 5 to 10 percent more people available and working in all or most of these categories.

Besides this huge army of professional, skilled, and semi-skilled health workers, the United States in 1970 had about 7,100 hospitals containing more than 1.6 million beds. On an average day in 1970, there were 1.3 million patients in American hospitals; for the entire year there were almost 32 million hospital admissions. Between 1960 and 1970 the number of persons in the United States rose only about 13 percent but the number of hospital admissions jumped by almost 27 percent. To serve their patients, American hospitals in 1970 employed more than 2.5 million people. The latter figure was about 1 million workers more than in 1960 and it averaged almost two hospital employees per hospital patient.

In the early 1970s Americans were getting not only more, but also better medical care than ever before. The improved quality reflected both the rapid recent gains in medical knowledge and the speed with which many of these advances have been introduced into practice. In 1970, the number of patient-physician contacts exceeded 1 billion by a comfortable margin. In an average week in the early 1970s, these data suggest there were 20 million or more patient-doctor contacts and about 2 million people spent at least one night in a hospital.

In the United States in the 1970s medical care is available to the great bulk of the population; it is not limited to a small clique of the rich and powerful. Nor is use of the most modern knowledge and the most expensive and elaborate therapeutic techniques available only to an affluent few. As this is written, for example, the world's longest-lived recipient of a heart transplant is a Negro, Louis Russell, an Indianapolis high school teacher who has survived for over four years with a stranger's heart in his chest. Mr. Russell's personal resources were certainly inadequate to pay for the superlative and enormously expensive operation and postoperative care he received.

There was a time in an earlier United States when millions of poor people had only charity medicine available to them and when moderately serious illness threatened bankruptcy for the middle class. But in the United States of the early 1970s there is less financial barrier to needed medical care than ever before. The legislative revolution of 1965 produced Medicare which now pays billions of dollars in medical bills annually for those sixty-five and over, and Medicaid which finances medical care for the poor. Moreover, the working class and the middle class have made giant strides toward assuring themselves of the financial means to cope with illness. In 1940 only 12 million Americans were covered by medical insurance. At the end of 1970, more than 170 million Americans under sixty-five had hospital insurance either from Blue Cross or from private insurance companies. Almost 160 million had insurance against surgical expenses and more than 136 million had insurance against nonsurgical medical costs. In addition, some 76 million Americans were covered by major medical insurance policies which provided financial protection beyond their limited first-level insurance policies. In 1970 these insurance plans paid out about $14.5 billion, including $9.3 billion for hospital expenses, almost $5 billion for doctors' bills and $200 million for dental expenses.[1]

Nor do Medicare, Medicaid, and private insurance exhaust the sources of medical care funds to supplement or replace direct payment by recipients of medical services. All members of the armed forces receive government-financed medical care, as do their dependents. Such care is also provided for veterans of the armed forces, who are treated in the large Veterans Administration medical centers. Nor should one forget the system of neighborhood health centers set up by the Office of Economic Opportunity and the Department of Health, Education, and Welfare. The consequence of all these measures is that in the United States today only a little more than one dollar out of every three spent on personal health expenditures is paid directly by the recipient of the services involved. The bulk of payment comes from third parties: the government, insurance companies, etc.

Much of this change has occurred only in the past few years. As recently as 1965, more than half of all personal health expenditures were paid directly by recipients. The point of all this can be stated very simply: In the United States today most medical care is paid for in such a way that the recipient sees it as totally or partially free and he has no feeling that the social security taxes or insurance premiums he pays are affected by whether he and his family have much or little medical care.[2]

Not all medical services appear equally "free" in the United States. In fiscal year 1970, individual direct payments accounted for less than one-sixth of all payments to hospitals. At the other extreme were drugs and medical appliances, 90 percent of whose cost was met by direct payment. Intermediate were the payments to physicians, dentists, and other suppliers of professional health services. About 55 percent of all these payments came directly from those receiving these professionals' services. Thus, to most Americans, hospital care seems most nearly "free" by a wide margin, followed by doctors' and dentists' services, while drugs and appliances are still paid for almost entirely by the actual consumers.

There is a growing body of opinion that the usual analyses of American medicine's problems put the cart before the horse, that the essence of the problem is not a doctor shortage but a patient surplus; that far from being too expensive, as is usually charged, American medical care is too cheap, at least in the eyes of the many who appear at doctors' offices and hospital doors expecting others to pay all or much of their bills. Here is the way Dr. Sidney Garfield, founder of the Kaiser-Permanente prepaid group medical plan, has put the matter:

> The cause of today's medical care crisis has been the inexorable spread of free care. The effect is an expanded and altered demand that is incompatible with the existing sick-care delivery system— wasting its medical manpower and threatening the quality and economics of the service it renders. . . . That result should not surprise anyone. Picture what would happen to air transportation if fares were eliminated and travel became a right. What chance would you have of getting any place if you really needed to? Even the highly automated telephone service would be staggered by removal of fees; necessary calls would become practically impossible. The change from fee to free would disrupt any system, no matter how well organized, and this is particularly true of medicine with its highly personalized sick-care service.[3]

Much discussion of the demand for medical care tends to focus on the technical and scientific advances which have so radically increased the potential usefulness of this care in preventing, alleviating, or curing illness. The importance of these factors is undeniable. But demand is greatly stimulated because many consumers see that they need bear no additional cost or relatively little cost to receive an additional unit of medical care. In this situation it would be remarkable if demand did not increase and increase radically. The more patients feel uninhibited by cost considerations from increasing their demands on the medical system, the more pressure they bring to bear on physicians who find increasingly that society is expecting them to exercise the control function formerly performed by costs and prices.

But the more the physician seeks to exercise this restraint, the more he risks antagonizing his patients and losing their patronage to other doctors who are more willing to let "free" medical care be exploited generously. Yet medical care is always expensive—and certainly never free—from society's point of view. It involves the use of highly trained and scarce personnel, as well as capital in the form of hospitals, X-ray machines, and other equipment.

In the field of medical costs, Americans today have the greatest amount of protection against the cost of a stay in the hospital. Hence it is hospital care that comes closest to seeming completely free. People with Blue Cross or other hospital insurance often do not have to make out-of-pocket payments until after 30, 120, or some other specified number of days of hospital residence have passed. Inevitably they try to receive as much of their medical care as possible in hospitals. The classic case involves diagnostic tests which can be administered on an ambulatory basis either in a physician's office or a hospital outpatient clinic. There are also marginal situations in which a patient has some degree of illness and the doctor must decide whether to leave him at home—where he can be taken care of at the cost of some inconvenience to the patient's family—or to send him to the hospital and thus free the family of all inconvenience as well as financial responsibility. The pressures on physicians in these cases can become very severe. Relatively few patients and their families care about the $60–$100 a day cost of semiprivate hospital accommodations as long as Blue Cross or a private insurance company or the government pays the bill. As a result, insurance companies and government medical agencies are deluged with bills for nonessential hospital services. The response of insurance company and government officials is a frantic effort to find devices to prevent patients from abusing "free" hospital care. Such devices are never as effective as was the original requirement that the patient who uses a hospital bed must pay for it.

Moreover, the lower the financial barriers to medical care, the greater the opportunity for abuse by those whom Dr. Garfield has termed the "worried well." Every practicing doctor knows there is a large group of persons in the population who come in frequently with varied and puzzling symptoms but who have nothing organically wrong with them so far as physical examination, chemical tests, X-ray examinations, and other diagnostic procedures can show. Anxiety and emotional distress can cause the widest range of symptoms, from gastric upset and headache to paralysis. Hypochondria has always been taken for granted among the wealthy to whom medical costs have never been a barrier. But as third party payers have taken over the medical costs of an ever larger fraction of the population, new and abundant opportunities have been created for less affluent hypochondriacs whose number is far from negligible.

Finally, the increasing spread of third party payment means that the struggles over medical costs are removed from the confrontation of physician and patient or hospital and patient. To the extent that medical costs are paid by the government from general tax revenues, the level of those costs becomes a factor in the unpleasant business of levying the general level of taxes. Understandably, congressmen became very upset when they discovered in the late 1960s that Medicare and Medicaid were costing much more than originally expected. State legislatures and governors have found themselves in the same unhappy position over Medicaid, and desperate efforts to cut escalating Medicaid costs now regularly spark angry political struggles in New York, California, and other states. The spiralling costs of medical insurance in recent years have produced anguish among all who have to pay them, whether employers or union members or both. Impassioned calls to keep medical costs from rocketing have come regularly from both business executives and union leaders. Union officials are dismayed by rising medical costs even where contracts provide for employer payment of all the bill. The union officials know that at the end of a hard-fought negotiation or strike there will be a finite sum for contract improvements. The larger the portion of this limited gain that has to go for paying higher medical insurance rates, the smaller the portion union members will receive in the visible and popular form of increased money wages. Thus top businessmen and union officials tend to have a common grudge against the medical system. Yet they seldom seem aware of their own contribution toward higher medical costs and overutilization of scarce medical resources, the contributions flowing from arrangements that make so much of medical care seem "free" to its recipients.

Inevitably, the fact that so much of American medical care is "free" or partly "free" encourages the belief that all medical care should be "free." People who take it for granted that a tuneup and major overhaul of their automobile will cost $100 or more are incensed when a physician charges $50–$60 for a physical checkup which includes a chest X-ray and various relevant laboratory tests. People who think nothing of spending $8–$10 for a bottle of liquor they will consume in a few days become angry when a week's supply of an antibiotic to cure an illness costs the same amount.

From this attitude it is but a short step to the assertion

that medical care is an inalienable human right that should be freely available to all. The political attractiveness of this idea has assured it substantial support inside and outside of Congress, especially from those who have not considered the costs and problems such a policy must bring in its wake.

The usual argument, of course, is that medical care is so important that it is immoral to leave it to the vagaries of the market place or to deny it to anyone because he is poor or a member of a disadvantaged minority or lives in some remote place. It would be difficult to disagree with this argument if medical care were the essential foundation of good health and if every visit to a physician or a hospital involved the saving of a human life. But any such notion is absurd.

An individual's health derives from many factors besides medical care. It depends upon his genetic endowment, his good luck in being born without birth injuries, his level of nutrition, his access to sanitary living conditions, and his willingness to exercise his body and avoid excesses such as drug addiction and alcoholism. Benjamin Franklin, for example, lived to be eighty-four years old in the eighteenth century when virtually the entire armamentarium of modern medical care was unknown. He was by no means unique; many other persons also reached old age in the centuries before antibiotics, anesthesia, kidney transplants, and other weapons of modern medicine were available. Their survival testified that the human body is equipped with effective natural defenses against illness, defenses developed during the long eons of evolution that produced modern man.

Such afflictions of today's American poor as wretched housing, rat bites, lead poisoning of their children, and hunger are not caused by lack of medical care. They require fundamental solutions beyond those that are taught in medical schools. Obviously a physician can help promote good health among young and middle-aged people by providing immunizations against some diseases, by supplementing the body's defenses against infection with pharmaceuticals, by patching up the victims of automobile and other accidents, and by keeping his eye out for such genetic diseases as juvenile diabetes and sickle cell anemia. But in these age groups, adequate nutrition, sanitary housing, avoidance of drug abuse and alcoholism, and the like are usually more important for good health than are the efforts of physicians. The notion of health care as a "right" that should be freely available in unlimited amounts makes sense only if one assumes society has infinite resources. But that assumption is false, and society must make hard choices about how to use limited resources. For most poor people, aid in satisfying their nonmedical needs is usually more important than an equivalent expenditure on medical facilities for them.

It is little understood that a very large fraction of the services provided by doctors each year have much more to do with comfort, convenience, and reassurance than with saving lives. The public discussion of medical care focuses upon cancer, heart disease, stroke, and other dread ailments. But much of the daily work of physicians deals with tension headaches, upset stomachs, colds, acne, or simply vague feelings of discomfort that often have no demonstrable organic basis. Most physical ailments, it is worth remembering, are self-limiting and will pass without a physician's ministrations. In the judgment of many physicians, the majority of the patients they see either have no organic sickness or have a minor illness for which medical attention is unnecessary. What many patients really come to a doctor for is reassurance, elementary psychiatric care or even—for the many lonely people in modern impersonal urban society—for simple human companionship. Many people go to a doctor today for help on matters that in a less atheistic age they would have taken to their priest or rabbi. Perhaps the highest praise many people can give their doctor is the proud statement, "He listens to my troubles," implying that his value is that he knows the patient and that he cares. It is difficult to believe that society is obligated to provide highly trained and scarce physicians to meet these needs without any cost to the patient. And to the extent that society permits the lonely, the hypochondriacal, and the mildly neurotic to occupy physician time needlessly as well as to take countless unnecessary chemical, X-ray and other tests—all at little or no immediate cost to the recipient—society wastes resources and diverts scarce manpower and facilities away from the treatment of those who are genuinely ill.

Some interesting evidence has been published recently to support the belief that the run of the mill, most frequent physician-patient meetings involve primarily symptomatic relief and medication designed to calm patients. The evidence comes from the Kaiser-Permanente San Francisco outpatient pharmacy list of the most frequently prescribed medications. This pharmacy is where Kaiser-Permanente patients—who pay very little or nothing extra to see a physician—go to get their drugs. Kaiser-Permanente researchers have made public the twenty-eight pharmaceuticals dispensed more than five hundred times from July 1 to September 30, 1969 at this pharmacy. The fifteen most frequently dispensed drugs are listed below, together with the frequency and the main use of each drug: [4]

Pharmaceutical	No. of Prescriptions	Chief Use
Darvon Compound	1,841	Pain relief
Donnatal	1,657	Stomach soother
Tetrachel	1,623	Antibiotic
Aspirin, phenacetin, caffeine, and codeine	1,511	Pain relief
Phenobarbitol	1,396	Sedative, tranquilizer
Librium	1,331	Tranquilizer
Miltown	1,225	Tranquilizer
Triamcinolone ointment	1,129	Anti-inflammatory salve
Penicillin G potassium	1,066	Antibiotic
Actifed	1,052	Decongestant
Esidrix	1,024	Diuretic
Valium	943	Tranquilizer
Reserpine	896	Tranquilizer, antihypertensive
Ferrous sulfate	866	Iron
Darvon	825	Pain relief

The large role of drugs for pain relief, sedation, and tranquilization in this list, along with an iron supplement and a decongestant, suggests that a substantial percentage of ailments for which these prescriptions were written were minor, self-limiting, or purely imaginary. They hardly seem like illnesses about which it would be worth exerting great passion, especially since over the counter, non-prescription medications—and perhaps even placeboes in many cases —could accomplish many of the same "therapeutic" goals. There is no reason to suppose that the pattern of minor or trivial complaints implied by this list of prescriptions differs from the pattern of practice experienced by other physicians engaged in primary care. Reassurance, we may suspect, was the chief contribution the Kaiser-Permanente physicians made to their patients' welfare. Once we realize that most people are basically healthy and that their complaints will disappear with the passage of time or after reassurance of some kind we can understand why there are people who swear by chiropractors, Christian Science readers, naturopaths, and other unorthodox purveyors of help. The continued economic viability of these non-medical practitioners would be impossible if their patrons did not feel they were helped. Probably the reported efficacy of many forms of traditional medicine, including acupuncture, in numerous countries over the centuries has a similar explanation.

At the other extreme from the hypochondriacs are the large numbers of people who become seriously ill each year and who do need extensive medical service. The proper care of such people will be expensive in any medical system because so much needs to be done for them. Unlike those who suffer from some minor ailment, they cannot be treated merely by providing symptomatic relief or by prescribing an antibiotic to combat infection.

The physician's first problem is that of diagnosis. This can be extremely complex in any patient with several symptoms, for two reasons: First, the range of possibilities is wide since the human organism can be prey to thousands of different diseases, either individually or in combination with each other. It is not uncommon, for example, for a patient to suffer simultaneously from, say, heart disease, diabetes, and cancer, or from some more esoteric combination of serious ailments. Second, real-life illnesses often manifest themselves in more complex fashion than the clearcut patterns of signs and symptoms listed in medical textbooks. Each human being is unique with individual variations in anatomy, biochemistry, and, often, the way in which a serious disease manifests itself.

Diagnosis is still an art, not an exact science. The physician attempts to determine what is wrong through physical examination of the patient, through study of the patient's past health history and through various tests which may help clear up the mysteries posed by the patient's condition. Some tests are chemical, based on analysis of the patient's blood, urine, or feces. Others involve analyzing the electrical discharges that accompany the operation of the heart and the brain, as in the electrocardiogram and the electroencephalogram. Many parts of the body can be probed by use of X-ray or radioactive isotopes or by sound waves. Thin tubes with lighted tips can be inserted into the body's orifices to look directly at the upper and lower ends of the gastrointestinal system, at the genitourinary system, at the upper end of the respiratory system. If necessary, surgery is resorted to and the appropriate part of the body is opened to examine the condition of the organs involved and to obtain samples of tissue for analysis (biopsy).

For diagnostic or therapeutic purposes several specialists may have to be called in, since no one physician has all the knowledge and skills to investigate, diagnose, and treat all diseases. Depending on the problem a cardiologist may be asked to study the heart, a nephrologist to ponder the kidney, or an endocrinologist to consider problems of hormonal and glandular function. The patient may have to be sent to an ear, nose, and throat specialist for examination of the bronchial passages with a bronchoscope, to a proctologist for a direct inspection of the lower colon, or to a urologist for a cystoscopic view of the urinary tract. For a complex X-ray, it may be necessary to get a specialist in heart catheterization. If exploratory surgery is needed, the appropriate specialist must be called in, a neurosurgeon if the brain or spinal cord is to be examined, a thoracic surgeon for the chest, an abdominal surgeon for that region, etc. And when tissue is removed, judgments about it must be made by highly trained and experienced pathologists. Is a tumor benign or malignant? For hundreds of thousands of Americans each year, that last question is the most momentous they have ever faced.

Once the diagnosis is established, the effort to treat the patient begins. At the simplest extreme this may involve only the administration of drugs or a relatively simple operation such as an appendectomy. At the other extreme it may involve a heart or kidney transplant whose execution requires a large team of physicians and technicians and whose success also demands extensive postoperative care to guard against infection and rejection of the transplanted organ or tissue. Very sick patients may be put into intensive care units and connected with machines that constantly monitor their heartbeat and other functions, machines that are always watched by specially trained nurses or doctors prepared to take instant action if something goes wrong. A patient who would otherwise die can be kept alive by putting him on a respirator which helps him to breathe or by using other equipment which performs vital functions that his disease-wracked body is temporarily unable to perform for itself.

Why is all this elaborate and expensive assembly of specialists, trained nurses and technicians, costly equipment, and the rest necessary? Without such resources many people would die much sooner than they now do, or else suffer permanent disabilities that can now be avoided or alleviated.

This elaborate organization and division of labor is at once the glory and the curse of American medicine. It is the glory because it has made routine many medical and surgical therapeutic feats which seem miraculous by the

standards of even a decade ago. It is the curse because it
has made medicine and medical care far more complex and
far more expensive than ever before, with resultant patient
and community dissatisfaction. The worst aspect of the
matter, of course, is that even the most prestigious and the
best medical staff using the finest available facilities cannot
guarantee success. Patients still die though they are treated
by teams of dedicated and highly trained physicians and
nurses, and if they die leaving large bills to be paid, the
anger and bitterness of the survivors have a special dimen-
sion. Yet even those who are helped and given, in effect, a
new lease on life all too often forget how sick and close to
death they were. They often complain about "greedy doctors" when the bills are presented. Often these are the same
people whose families—at the time of crisis—implored the
physicians to "spare no expense" and "call in any consul-
tant from anywhere" to save the sick relative. It is common
knowledge that many patients or former patients are angry
at those they view as inconsiderate or grasping doctors. It is
less well understood that many physicians are equally unhappy about ungrateful patients, some of whom simply
walk off without paying their bills, regardless of what has
been done for them.

Because of the awesome complexity of the human organism, medicine is still often an art, an imprecise undertaking
in which the physician's intuition, clinical judgment, and
experience play as much of a role as purely scientific procedures. The patient recites his complaints and his medical
history; the physician performs a physical examination and
formulates a tentative hypothesis or clinical impression; the
hypothesis is tested by reference both to the patient's subse-
quent progress and to the new information gained from laboratory, X-ray and other examinations. As noted earlier,
the body can be prey to thousands of illnesses, singly or in

combination. Its mechanisms for showing that something is wrong are limited. Any individual symptom may have many possible meanings. Thus a headache may reflect nothing more than simple nervous tension, or it may be a sign of a fatal brain tumor; slight fever and nausea may be the result of a mild 24–hour virus or the first signs of any one of a dozen potentially fatal infections. Faced by this problem every day and in every case, the physician has no choice but to play the game of probabilities. He knows that the mildest diseases are the commonest and that the crippling or fatal ailments are uncommon, even extremely rare. Therefore, pondering a set of signs and symptoms, his first working hypothesis is usually that they are the product of some common and not too dangerous disease, but he tries to maintain a high index of suspicion. The initial hypothesis is subject to rapid change if the symptoms persist and / or the patient's condition grows worse. (When the patient exhibits initial symptoms that are life threatening, of course, the physician reacts energetically immediately.)

As he considers each patient's complaints and seeks to formulate diagnosis and therapy, the physician finds himself always between Scylla and Charybdis. He may err by underestimating an ailment, failing to get enough information about the patient, and then finding to his surprise that he has a very sick person on his hands. The potential costs of this kind of error are primarily the suffering and danger experienced by the patient, but they also include the psychological blow to the physician, the damage to his reputation among those familiar with the case, and—increasingly, these days—the burden of a malpractice suit charging the physician with negligence responsible for a patient's suffering or death.

It might seem at first sight as though there were an easy

way to avoid these troubles. The physician might adopt the policy of taking every patient's complaint in the most serious light possible and treating every set of symptoms as the onset of a fatal or permanent crippling disease. But to do so is to fall into the second kind of error. For such an attitude means the physician orders many of his patients into the hospital needlessly, keeps them away from work for relatively long periods, and subjects them to numerous unnecessary laboratory, X-ray, radioactive isotope, and other tests. This kind of behavior immediately drives up the cost of medical care substantially and raises the possibility that the patient may be hurt rather than helped. The latter possibility arises, of course, because many clinical tests involve risks and potential health costs. Any X-ray examination adds to the recipient's radiation burden and increases the small but nonetheless real possibility of genetic damage to the patient's progeny as well as of radiation-induced cancer. There is also a small but real risk of serious injury or death in such procedures as renal biopsy, heart catheterization, and the like. Finally, of course, the physician who treats every cough as a sign of tuberculosis and every neck swelling as lymphoma will soon get a reputation for trying to exploit his patients by overdoctoring them so he can collect more and larger fees.

Thus in every case the physician faces the prospect of being damned if he does and damned if he doesn't. The goal of both his classroom and his clinical training is to give him the ability to walk the tightrope between underdoctoring and overdoctoring. But physicians do not practice in a vacuum; they are subject to the powerful societal forces working on them all the time and these forces push in different directions. The media, insurance companies, and government officials concerned with Medicare and

Medicaid complain loudly and bitterly about how expensive medical care is and how important it is to cut down on hospitalization, on unnecessary tests, and the like. But the physician also knows that the number of malpractice suits, the size of awards in these suits, and the cost of his annual malpractice insurance premium are increasing. Should he order that extra blood test or X-ray examination or specialist consultation if he knows there is only one chance in twenty that the patient will gain anything from the additional effort? Should he order the additional test or consultation if the chance of gain is only one in one hundred or one in one thousand? Inevitably, these days, fear of a malpractice suit will play a role in the decision, with the result that medical care costs more than it should. The physician who does not practice such "defensive medicine" knows that he and his insurance company could pay heavily for that failure and that at the extreme he might be forced out of practice by the inability to have malpractice insurance at all. If patients had to pay out of their own pockets immediately for all the extra hospitalization, the extra tests, and the extra consultations physicians prescribe out of fear of malpractice suits, they would exert useful pressure for economizing. But where these costs are mainly paid for by medical insurance or the government, patients have little incentive to protest precautions taken against even very unlikely risks.

The potentials in all this became dramatically visible in 1970–1971 after the Blue Cross-Blue Shield policies for federal government employees were revised to include out-of-hospital diagnostic tests as a fully paid benefit. The huge and unexpected expansion in demand for these tests was the major factor in rolling up a deficit of almost 16 million dollars for this Blue Cross-Blue Shield program in 1971.

Typically in this situation, Blue Cross-Blue Shield officials felt they could not afford to ask federal employees to give up the benefit, so the two organizations asked for a 34.1 percent increase in premiums. That request stirred up a storm of protests which did not end when the Price Commission ordered that the increase be cut to 22 percent.

There are many theories as to why malpractice suits have become an increasingly serious factor in American medical care and practice in recent years. Many physicians tend to blame it all on the system of contingency fees for lawyers common in these cases. This, they believe, encourages allegedly rapacious lawyers who search out potential clients and who are willing to initiate many unsuccessful suits because one court victory can be so profitable. Malpractice specialists among attorneys, not unnaturally, reply in a similarly angry spirit, arguing that the increasingly sophisticated patient is less willing to assume the doctor is always right regardless of the outcome of a case. An intermediate view holds that the greater demands on the American medical system and the growing specialization of physicians are both making for increasingly depersonalized care.

Whatever the truth of these theories, they do suggest it is worthwhile to look at the current organization of American medicine, one of the key factors involved in determining how personal or impersonal care may be today. At the end of 1971, according to the American Medical Association, there were 287,248 M.D.'s involved in patient care. Of these somewhat less than 10 percent, 23,518, were federal government employees, presumably physicians working for the armed forces, the Veterans Administration, the Public Health Service, and for special government health care delivery projects. The remainder, 263,730, were either in private practice, employees of state and municipal governments or of non-medical corporations, or hospital employees. The distribution of these 263,730 physicians was as follows:

Interns	11,460
Residents	36,977
Hospital-employed attending physicians	20,361
Physicians in office-based practice	194,932

Most American physicians are solo practitioners working on a fee for service basis. They are independent entrepreneurs who see patients and charge fees for the services performed. Most often each physician has his own office or shares an office with one or several other doctors; usually, he employs a receptionist and frequently, one or more registered or practical nurses as well as one or more technicians or assistants. Many physicians have modest laboratory facilities for the most common tests as well as X-ray equipment and machines to take electrocardiograms and other standard measures of body function. For a large fraction of the ailments that send people to a doctor's office, the equipment in the average general practitioner's, internist's, or pediatrician's office is quite adequate.

The critics who paint the picture of the typical American physician as an isolated artisan doing as he pleases and tackling the most varied tasks, even those he is incompetent to handle, exaggerate grossly, however. There are such instances, of course, particularly in the case of an isolated physician in a small town or other sparsely settled area. But normally a physician is a member of a large, informal medical community that has been called "a group without walls." Such an informal group consists of a number of physicians who cooperate and help each other without any written contract or other agreement. Some of the cooperation involves one physician taking over another's practice while the latter is ill or on vacation or simply taking a weekend or night off. Such informal groups normally include both primary physicians and specialists, the latter being the doctors to whom the former refer their patients when they feel consultation is needed. Normally, but not always, a physician also has hospital admitting privileges and does some of his practice in cooperation with other physicians in the hospital or hospitals at which he treats his more seriously ill patients. Where several physicians share an office, the chances are good that they at least will constitute such an informal group. In many communities the practice is increasingly that of having one or more community medical buildings in which both primary physicians and specialists have their offices so that consultations, the more complicated laboratory or X-ray examinations, and other supplementary services can be provided with a minimum of inconvenience to the patient. The details of how medical care is provided vary from physician to physician and from community to community.

The system that now exists is inevitably complex. Moreover, it does not work perfectly by any means, as evidenced by complaints from patients who are unable to get doctors at night or on weekends, or from patients who have had to travel long distances and lose much time going from one physician to another or from a physician's office to a testing laboratory. Those who stress such complaints—which should not be ignored—forget that there are millions of patients who do not complain because they have access to doctors when they need them and because they do not have to travel far from a primary physician to a specialist or a laboratory. Unfortunately those who are well served tend literally to be a silent majority.

Like any other small entrepreneur, the solo practitioner lives or dies economically by how well he satisfies his customers, in this case his patients. The fee for service provides the monetary incentive to do a good job, to be available when needed, and to cultivate a good reputation both for ability and for personality. The solo practitioner in a medium-sized or large community knows that he has no monopoly, that his patient can go elsewhere if he is displeased. This adds to the doctor's incentive to do his best. Like all human arrangements, this system can be abused and some critics charge that solo practitioners working on a fee for service basis tend to subject their patients to unnecessary surgery or otherwise overdoctor them in order to gain more fees. But at the same time it is charged that there is an acute doctor shortage and that every physician has more work than he can handle. The two accusations are hardly consistent since a doctor who is overworked and has patients storming his doors has no incentive to overdoctor them in any way. The truth is that all kinds of situations exist and that there are cases both of overdoctoring and underdoctoring. But the threat of malpractice suits and of condemnation by other physicians tends to discourage abuses, though some abuses do occur. There is no reason to suppose that most physicians are any less honorable than other men and any less anxious to do an honest and capable job. The great majority of sick Americans who consult physicians are helped. Many are cured and others have their discomfort eased, though there are ailments against which medicine has no weapons. Many patients come for emotional support and reassurance and it is the fee for service practitioner, anxious for his patient's good will, who is least likely to dispense impersonal care.

Solo practitioners are not the only element of American

medicine. In 1969, the AMA reports, this country had some 6,371 formally organized groups of three or more physicians. These group arrangements included more than forty thousand physicians, or roughly one in five of all American physicians who had completed their residency training and were engaged in patient care. Two-thirds of these groups were small three- or four-doctor partnerships, some of them single specialty groups, say, all dermatologists or all radiologists; others were multispecialty groups combining, say, internists, surgeons, and gynecologists. At the other extreme were 147 groups—including almost 9,-500 doctors—each of which included more than twenty-five physicians. Most groups of physicians operate on a fee for service basis, but in 1969 there were 396 groups which provided some or all of their services on a prepaid basis. There were only 85 groups, however, which provided more than half of the medical care they dispensed on a prepaid basis. The most famous and largest of these prepaid groups are those associated with the Kaiser-Permanente organizations in California, Oregon, Hawaii, Denver, and Cleveland but they are still the exception in the early 1970's. We shall have more to say about prepaid group practices later in this volume.

NOTES

1. Data from the Health Insurance Council's twenty-fifth annual survey of private health insurance coverage in the United States.
2. *Statistical Abstract of the United States 1971*, p. 62.
3. *Medical Group News and Health Services Report*, October 1971.
4. Gary D. Friedman *et al.*, "Experience in Monitoring Drug Reactions in Outpatients: The Kaiser-Permanente Drug Monitoring System," *Journal of the American Medical Association*, August 2, 1971, p. 569.

CHAPTER II

WHAT HEALTH CRISIS?

"By all measures, Americans are less healthy now than they were twenty years ago." That was the unhappy news the *Washington Post* presented to its readers on December 26, 1970, in an article by its medical reporter, Stuart Auerbach. If true, that statement would be the most damning possible indictment of the American medical system. In the twenty years before 1970, medical science progressed with unprecedented rapidity and some of those gains should have been translated into concrete health gains for the American people. It is some such dark evaluation of American medicine that must be in the minds of many who agitate for radical change and who use the terms "health care crisis" and "health crisis" interchangeably. Some similar image may have been in the mind of Thomas J. Watson, Jr. when—a week before Mr. Auerbach's article appeared—he wrote derisively of "our own U.S.A., the home of the free, the home of the brave, and the home of a decrepit, inefficient, high priced system of medical care." [1]

But the statement from the *Washington Post* quoted above was simply wrong. All persons familiar with the facts know that there has been enormous progress in improving the health of the American people since 1950. Ordinary, everyday observation as well as a mass of statistical data indicate that the great majority of Americans are indeed quite healthy physically, that a larger fraction of American babies survive the dangerous first year of life than ever before, and that unprecedented numbers of Americans are now surviving to their seventies, eighties, nineties, and even beyond the century mark. The dimensions of this progress are indicated by a government report to the White House Conference on Aging in late 1971. Since the previous such conference a decade earlier, the report noted, the United States population sixty-five years or older increased from 16.6 million to 20 million persons, roughly 10 percent of the total number of people in this country. For a longer range perspective, the report noted that between 1870 and 1970, when the nation's total population increased five times, the number of persons sixty-five years or older rose seventeen times.[2]

The improved health of the American people has been a basic factor making possible this country's increasing population and rise in average longevity. These gains in turn have helped create contemporary concern about overpopulation and the ecological threat of continued expansion in the numbers and living standard of the nation's people. Ultimately, it is the decline in infant mortality and other forms of premature death that has produced today's movements for zero population growth, legalized abortion, and even euthanasia. There was no need for artificial population control when death from infectious diseases and other ailments claimed numerous victims each year from all age groups. Many of the great killers of the past were banished by such public health measures as the provision of pure water and pure milk, the sanitary disposition of sewage and garbage, and government inspection of food. The recent gains are partly attributable to the triumphs of modern medical science, from the discovery of hormone therapy and antibiotics to the emergence of today's advanced surgery. The growing affluence of American society has contributed to better health by making possible adequate nutrition and housing for most of the population. In turn these gains have intensified concern about the millions of Americans who do not share this affluence.

The nation's increased wealth has also had negative consequences. It has made possible the widespread use of automobiles which claim tens of thousands of accident victims annually. It has also made possible the life styles of the millions who are obese, sedentary in their habits and, therefore, prime candidates for heart disease. The medical system cannot justly be blamed for these features of modern civilization, nor for the homicides, the deaths due to narcotics addiction, or the war casualties which have accounted for such a large fraction of American deaths in the eighteen to forty year age bracket this past decade. Some observers even argue that medical care is overemphasized in the search for better public health, as in this statement by two Carnegie-Mellon University researchers:

An individual's general health status depends not only on his socioeconomic status but also on his life style and environment. His drinking, eating and exercising habits all influence his health, as does the environment in which he works and lives. It has been shown that air pollution leads to increases in the incidence of bronchitis, lung cancer, other respiratory diseases, and many other diseases. A recent study concluded that a fifty percent abatement in the level of air pollution would lower the economic cost of morbidity and mortality almost as much as finding an immediate and complete cure for cancer. For middle class families in cities, air pollution is probably the single most important factor adversely affecting family health. Relatively small expenditures on abating pollution would do more to improve the general health of the family than much larger expenditures on medical care that the family currently undertakes.[3]

Let us turn now to a more systematic evaluation of the nation's health. Perhaps the best single summary measure in this area is life expectancy at birth, a figure that changes annually with the changes in the age patterns of death each year. Here are the data summarizing the changes in American life expectancy at birth since 1930: [4]

Year	Total	White Male	White Female	Nonwhite Male	Nonwhite Female
		(life	expectancy	in	years)
1930	59.7	59.7	63.5	47.3	49.2
1940	62.9	62.1	66.6	51.5	54.9
1950	68.2	66.5	72.2	59.1	62.9
1960	69.7	67.4	74.1	61.1	66.3
1967	70.5	67.8	75.1	61.1	68.2
1970	70.8	*	*	*	*
1971	71.1	*	*	*	*

* Not available

On the average an American baby born in 1971 could expect to live 11.4 years longer than an American baby born in 1930. The most impressive gain was made by non-white females who could expect to live 19 years longer if they were born in 1967 than if they had been born in 1930. The second largest absolute gain was made by nonwhite males whose life expectancy rose almost 14 years between 1930 and 1967. The life expectancy of white females rose almost 12 years between 1930 and 1967, while that of white males increased 8.1 years. The magnitude of the achievement is spotlighted if we look at the percentage figures. Between 1930 and 1967, life expectation of a nonwhite female rose almost 40 percent, of a nonwhite male almost 30 percent, of a white female almost 20 percent, and of a white male almost 15 percent.

The data show also that there are significant differences among major groups in the United States population. Among both whites and nonwhites, females have substantially longer life expectancies than males. Looking at both sexes together, whites have a longer life expectancy than nonwhites, though nonwhite females had a slightly better life expectancy in 1967 than white males. The sources of these differences are partially biological—certainly as regards the female superiority to the male—and partially environmental, including such factors as the relative socioeconomic deprivation and poverty of nonwhites as compared with whites.

It has been argued that it is primarily the lack of access to medical care that explains the poorer health—including life expectancy—of nonwhites compared to whites. There is no disposition here to deny that improved medical care for nonwhites is desirable and could improve the statistical record shown above. But whether access to medical care is the key factor may be doubted. Presumably nonwhite females live under the same disadvantages as nonwhite males, yet the nonwhite females had a 7.1 year superiority in life expectancy to the males of that group. Though white males on the average presumably had better access to medical care than nonwhite females, the white males had a lower life expectancy.

The belief that environmental and socioeconomic factors are more important than access to medical care is strengthened by a recent study by the Public Health Service, which investigated the changing mortality rates of American males in the late 1950s and much of the 1960s. This study emphasized the rising importance of such causes of death as lung cancer, cirrhosis of the liver, homicide, suicide, and automobile accidents.[5]

Lung cancer deaths could be cut by a drastic reduction in cigarette smoking. Cirrhosis of the liver could be reduced if consumption of alcohol were cut sharply. The homicide death toll would probably be decreased most rapidly by action that would end the easy availability of guns. Automobile accidents and deaths could be slashed by a complex of measures ranging from the provision of better safety devices in motor cars to rigorous enforcement of laws prohibiting driving while under the influence of alcohol. In the latter area the precedent set by Sweden— where police patrols stop cars at random and test drivers to see whether they have recently ingested alcohol—could usefully be followed in this country. The reader will notice that all these techniques for improving the longevity of American males are nonmedical in character.

The second most frequently cited index of a nation's health is its infant mortality rate. Here, too, the United States data testify to impressive gains over both the long run and the short run. In 1930, 64.6 American babies out of every 1,000 live births died before the age of one year. Twenty years later, in 1950, that toll had been cut to less than half, to an infant mortality rate of 29.2. If that 1950 rate had continued unchanged, about 110,000 of the babies born in 1970 would have died before the age of one year. Happily, the infant mortality rate in 1970 was significantly lower than in 1950, an improvement that translated into the survival of 35,000 babies who would have died in 1970 if there had been no progress since 1950. A more detailed

statistical view of the pace of this improvement is shown
below: [6]

Year	Total	White	Nonwhite
	(*infant mortality per thousand live births*)		
1950	29.2	26.8	44.5
1960	26.0	22.9	43.2
1965	24.7	21.5	40.3
1970	19.8	17.4	31.4
1971	19.2	16.8	30.2
1972 *	18.6	16.2	29.0

* Estimated on basis of data for January–June 1972.

Two striking facts emerge from these data. One is the
very rapid decline of infant mortality rates since 1965, a
drop that contrasts particularly with the much slower improvement during 1950–1965. This was particularly true
of nonwhite infant mortality which declined twice as much
in 1965–1970 as it did in the previous fifteen years. The
second striking fact is the continuing great disparity between white and nonwhite infant mortality.

We can only speculate about the reasons for the relatively
spectacular fall in infant mortality after 1965. The emphasis on this indicator during the debate about proposed
changes in the medical system may have had some influence by sensitizing the medical profession and encouraging
energetic action to provide better facilities for critically ill
babies. Useful, too, was the spread of government-financed
comprehensive child care programs. Medicaid probably
played some role by making medical help more available to
poor people, especially pregnant women and babies in poor
families. The increased use of contraceptives and the increasing legalization of abortions in the late 1960s and the

early 1970s also helped lower infant mortality by reducing the number of babies born in high risk family environments. More than anything else, the sharp decline in nonwhite infant mortality after 1965 may well reflect the rapid improvement in income and education from which many black Americans benefited after the mid-1960s.

The white-nonwhite differential in infant mortality shown above is somewhat misleading. The highest infant mortality rates are experienced by blacks, American Indians, Puerto Ricans, and Chicanoes, though the latter two groups are classified as whites. The common denominators among these groups are the heavy tolls exacted by poverty and social disorganization. Among blacks, for example, the tragic toll of high infant mortality rates is related to the high incidence of illegitimate births, often to very young mothers who do not know how to care for themselves during pregnancy and who have inadequate knowledge and resources to care for their babies. The lowest rates of infant mortality are found among the middle and upper classes, including not only whites but also nonwhites. Japanese and Chinese in this country actually have very low infant mortality rates, probably a reflection of their economic welfare, educational levels and life styles rather than of anything to do with race or skin color. Infant mortality in this country, in short, is more a socioeconomic than a medical problem.

The low correlation between infant mortality and the availability of physicians can be demonstrated statistically. The table below shows the twelve states with lowest 1970 infant mortality rates, as well as the physician-population ratio and the percentage of Negroes in each state, the latter an approximate index of the relative importance of poor people in each state's population.[7]

	1970 *Infant* *Mortality*	1969 *Physicians /* *100,000 population*	1970 *Percent* *Negroes*
United States	19.8	163	11.2
North Dakota	14.1	97	0.4
Utah	15.3	137	0.6
Idaho	16.3	95	0.3
Massachusetts	16.4	214	3.1
Wisconsin	16.4	126	2.9
Connecticut	16.5	190	6.0
Minnesota	16.8	155	0.9
Oregon	16.9	152	2.1
Vermont	17.1	197	0.2
California	17.1	194	7.0
Maine	17.2	131	0.3
Nebraska	17.3	119	2.7

The lack of any close connection between the availability of physicians in a state and its infant mortality rate is plain in the data above. Two of the three states having the lowest infant mortality rates in the country also have among the lowest physician to population ratios in the nation, while Massachusetts, tied for fourth place, has one of the highest such ratios. All of the states in this top twelve have percentages of Negro population that are well below the national average. If we look at the other extreme, at the states with the highest infant mortality rates in 1970, we find most of them in the Deep South. These are states like Mississippi, Alabama, and Louisiana, which combine relatively high percentages of Negro population with relatively low physician to population ratios.

The data below give the same information as the preceding table for the five states with the highest infant mortality rates in 1970.

	1970 Infant Mortality	1969 Physicians / 100,000 population	1970 Percent Negroes
Mississippi	28.2	78	36.8
Louisiana	25.1	115	29.9
Alabama	24.3	86	26.4
North Carolina	23.9	107	22.4
Nevada	23.5	118	5.7

A comparison of these last two tables discloses a striking fact: North Dakota and Idaho, which had two of the lowest infant mortality rates in 1970, had fewer doctors in relation to population than Louisiana, North Carolina, and Nevada, three of the five states with the highest infant mortality rates that year. Once again we find evidence that under contemporary conditions in the United States health— more specifically here, infant mortality—and the medical system have only a low correlation, while nonmedical factors such as poverty, education, and lifestyle are probably more important.

A frequent indictment of American medicine derives from international comparisons, particularly the fact that some foreign nations have statistics showing higher life expectancy at birth and lower infant mortality rates than the United States. A relatively moderate statement of that indictment was given in the 1971 HEW White Paper on Health:

. . . the United States is not performing as well as other advanced nations. Our ranking as 13th in infant mortality rates is the key indicator of relatively poor performance. Even if all the statistical variations were straightened out, so that the rank of the United States rose to 11th or 10th, there would be little rejoicing. For the belief is that the United States, with its great abundance, should have the lowest infant death rate, and the expectations are that it can achieve that rank.

A full page in this "White Paper" is devoted to charts showing that the United States ranks not only 13th in infant mortality but 18th in male life expectancy and 11th in female life expectancy. The implication here and in other, usually less restrained, versions of this argument is that if only major changes were made in the organization and delivery of American medical care infant mortality and life expectancy in this country could be raised quickly to the best in the world. Yet we have already seen the sobering statistics that a number of the individual states having the fewest doctors available relative to population also have the lowest infant mortality.

The "White Paper" statement does take into account one basic problem that more politically oriented statements do not, namely the statistical difficulties in international comparisons. These arise because of differing definitions and degrees of completeness in the accounting of deaths and births in different countries. There are two additional basic weaknesses in this argument. One is the assumption that infant mortality and life expectancy in modern industrial nations are primarily dependent upon the amount and quality of medical care. The second fallacy is the assumption that the United States is really comparable with the countries that have seemingly better indices of health. Let us consider these matters in turn.

On the first issue, the arguments made earlier about the tenuous relation between medical care and infant mortality, life expectancy, etc., need not be repeated here. But it seems worthwhile to review some evidence from foreign sources that even in countries with fully socialized medical systems there are wide geographic differences in health because of nonmedical factors. The Soviet Union, for example, has recently published data on infant mortality rates in twenty-one of its largest cities. The data, given below, seem revealing: [8]

City	1970 Infant Mortality Rate
Dushambe	47
Tashkent	41
Ashkhabad	33
Alma Ata	27
Kuibyshev	27
Erevan	27
Frunze	26
Novosibirsk	25
Baku	24
Gorky	22
Sverdlovsk	22
Tbilisi	22
Moscow	21
Leningrad	20
Kharkov	20
Minsk	19
Kiev	18
Tallin	18
Kishinev	17
Vilnyus	15
Riga	15

This table immediately reveals the wide dispersion of urban infant mortality rates in the Soviet Union. Dushambe had three times as high a rate as Vilnyus and Riga. Moreover the cities with the worst infant mortality rates in the Soviet Union are primarily in Soviet Central Asia, i.e., they are cities with relatively large Moslem populations. And Soviet Moslems are not unlike Negroes in the United States in terms of relatively high birth rates, relative poverty, lack of education, and some other socioeconomic characteristics. The lowest Soviet urban infant mortality rates are in the most western Soviet republics which have very low birth rates and which were not annexed to the Soviet Union until 1941. These huge differences in infant mortality—so obviously connected with cultural and socioeconomic factors —persist in the Soviet Union despite the fact that country has a fully socialized medical system with nominally equal, "free" access to medical care for all. Moreover, if one wants to make comparisons with American cities, it is worth noting that the list above shows a half dozen major Soviet cities with infant mortality rates roughly equal to or above that of Washington, D.C., while the infant mortality rate of New York City is at the level of Moscow and Leningrad.

The same phenomenon of great diversity of infant mortality rates in a country with socialized medicine is visible in Britain. Here are the data for major areas of that country, which is smaller and much more homogenous than the Soviet Union.[9]

		Infant Mortality Rate
England and Wales		
	Urban	19.0
	Rural	16.0
Northern Ireland		
	Urban	25.4
	Rural	21.4
Scotland		
	Urban	22.6
	Rural	19.3

These data are for 1967. In that year urban Northern Ireland had an infant mortality rate that was 50 percent higher than in rural England and Wales, as well as substantially higher than in urban England and Wales and in urban Scotland.

Let us examine our second point: International comparisons can be misleading if made without consideration for the huge differences between individual countries with regard to their populations and life patterns. The critics of American medicine would rightly scoff at any comparison between United States infant mortality and life expectancy and those of India, yet they accept uncritically and trumpet loudly similarly defective comparisons in the opposite direction.

The United States is wealthy and industrialized. It is also a nation with a very large and heterogeneous population distributed over a vast continental area whose climatic conditions vary from the tropical and semitropical environments of Hawaii, Southern California, and Southern Florida to the harsh northern ambience of Alaska. Included in our population are representatives of almost every group of mankind from the Nordic blondes of Scandinavia to the swarthy peoples of the Mediterranean, the blacks of Africa, and many diverse peoples of Asia. Elsewhere in the world there is only one other large nation which is relatively affluent by world standards, highly industrialized, and composed of many heterogeneous population groups distributed over a continental area. This is the Soviet Union, a country with, as noted earlier, a completely socialized system of medical care.

The detractors of American medicine rarely compare United States data with that of the Soviet Union, at least in

48   THE CASE FOR AMERICAN MEDICINE

public. The reason is simple: With respect to life expectancy
at birth and infant mortality, United States health statistics
are superior to those of the Soviet Union. Below are the infant mortality rates of the two countries during the decade
1960–1969: [10]

Year	United States	Soviet Union
1960	26.0	35
1961	25.3	32
1962	25.3	32
1963	25.2	31
1964	24.8	29
1965	24.7	27
1966	23.7	26
1967	22.4	26
1968	21.8	26
1969	20.7	26

Despite the many similarities between the United States
and the Soviet Union, however, there are also many differences between them. Hence the above data cannot be
simplistically interpreted to mean that the private medical
system of the United States is necessarily superior to the socialized medical organization of the Soviet Union. Conversely, the data showing that the United States is 13th in
infant mortality among the nations of the world or 11th in
female life expectancy at birth do not show that the United
States medical system is inferior to that of other countries.
There are just too many nonmedical factors involved to
permit such simplified judgments.

Nevertheless it is worth looking somewhat more closely
at the world situation in infant mortality rates. The table
below shows these rates in 1960 and 1970 for a representative sample of the world's industrialized nations: [11]

Country	1960 1970 (infant mortality rates)		1970 Population (millions)
United States	26.0	19.8	205
Netherlands	16.5	12.7	13
Sweden	16.6	13.1*	8
Norway	18.7	13.7*	4
Australia	20.2	17.9	13
Switzerland	21.1	15.4**	6
United Kingdom	22.4	18.6**	56
Czechoslovakia	23.5	22.9**	14
Canada	27.3	19.3	22
France	27.5	15.1	51
Belgium	30.7	21.7	10
Japan	30.7	13.1	103
Israel	30.8	23.6	3
West Germany	33.8	23.5	60
Italy	43.8	29.2	54

* 1968   ** 1969

The population figures shown above provide an immediate warning against facile comparisons between the United States, with its more than 200,000,000 people, and such small nations as the Netherlands, Sweden, and Norway which all together have only little more than 10 percent as many people as the United States. Beyond that basic fact, these data show how diverse international experience in reducing infant mortality was between 1960 and 1970. All the countries listed made progress, but their gains were highly unequal and there are no obvious or easy reasons for these differences. Japan, whose rapid industrialization in the 1960s made it a world power again, registered the most impressive progress. Czechoslovakia, despite its fully socialized system of medical care, made the smallest gain over the decade. And where Czechoslovakia had been appreciably ahead of the United States in 1960, it was appreciably behind as the decade ended. The United States, which recorded about a 25 percent decline in infant mortality over the decade, performed roughly as well percentagewise as most of the industrialized nations. In short, it is hard to read the statistics about infant mortality as proving anything very clearcut about the disadvantages or advantages of different systems of medical care. What the data do suggest is that it is highly homogenous nations— like Japan, Sweden, and the Netherlands—that are now registering the best records in saving the lives of infants. The argument that it is somehow only the deficiencies of the private practice of medicine that explain this country's ranking in the infant mortality sweepstakes can seem persuasive only to the statistically unsophisticated.

The discussion to this point has emphasized infant mortality and life expectancy at birth as indicators of community health. For a wider view we must turn to the specific diseases which have historically been the great killers and causes of disability, diseases such as bubonic plague, smallpox, cholera, diphtheria, typhoid, and typhus. They were once extremely serious in this country; today they are either completely unknown or they strike so few victims annually that they are medical and statistical curiosities. Tuberculosis, once a great killer of poor Americans, black and white alike, still persists, but its incidence is far lower than in past years when a much less populous United States took it for granted that each year there would be hundreds of thousands of new tuberculosis cases. Millions of older Americans still remember vividly the annual polio epidemics and scares that began each spring; today's "now" generation knows polio only as something mentioned in the history books. Measles, too, has recently joined the ranks of almost-vanquished diseases as a new vaccine has saved millions of children from the discomfort and danger of an actual attack.

Much of the progress toward preventing these infectious diseases was made before and during World War II. But even in the 1960s there were important additional gains in this country. The data below show the decline in reported cases of some of these diseases between 1960 and 1971.[12]

Disease	Number of Cases Reported	
	1960	1971
Diphtheria	918	202
Measles	441,703	75,007
Whooping cough	14,809	3,036
Polio	3,190	12
Tuberculosis*	55,494	35,035
Typhoid fever	816	415

* Newly reported active cases.

For an even more dramatic picture of the health revolution that has taken place this century in the United States, let us look at how death rates from common infectious diseases have plunged since 1900.[13]

Cause of Death	1900	1940	1970
	(Deaths per 100,000 population)		
Diarrhea	142.7	10.3	1.1
Measles	13.3	0.5	0.1
Diphtheria	40.3	1.1	0.0
Whooping cough	12.2	2.2	0.0
Dysentery	12.0	1.9	0.1
Tuberculosis	194.4	45.8	2.7
Pneumonia	202.2	70.1	28.6

The truly historic gains depicted in these figures reflect the impact of improved public health measures, higher living standards, and the availability of antibiotics and immunizing vaccines. By the standards of today, there was certainly a health crisis in 1900, and even in 1940.

Against this background particularly, the question recurs of how one can seriously speak of a health crisis in the early 1970s. Perhaps the kindest answer is to refer to the revolution of rising expectations. A population exposed to incessant publicity—most of it quite correct—about the miracles of modern medicine takes for granted the enormous progress of the past and even of the present and wonders why anyone should be sick, or even why anyone should die. What is not accepted, apparently, is the fact that all human beings are mortal and that medicine can only hope to prolong life for some finite period. Millions who, in an earlier era, would have died of tuberculosis, pneumonia, smallpox, or other infectious diseases are now saved to die of heart disease, cancer, and stroke.

Additionally, the very successes of medicine create new problems. Many people with genetic defects who would have died at an early age in previous epochs now survive to become adults, to procreate and pass their defective genes on to the next generation. There is much talk about genetic counseling and advising young people with potentially lethal genes not to have children, but how effective is this in reality? Questions are being raised about the consequences of this reproduction for the future of the human genetic pool and some pessisimists have suggested the need for coercion to prevent, say, hemophiliacs and juvenile diabetics, among others, from having children. Difficult political struggles over such issues could arise in the future. Already some Negro sources have denounced as "genocide" efforts to warn persons having the genetic endowment for sickle-cell anemia against marrying each other and having children. Sickle-cell anemia is a disease afflicting blacks almost exclusively.

The successes of medicine have meant and will continue to mean that increasing numbers of people will survive into the older age brackets. Today many of these survivors are the victims of long term degenerative illnesses whose proper care is extremely expensive. Many of them, too, survive long after their spouses and in some cases even their children have died, leaving them alone and often without adequate economic resources. Finally, of course, even the sickest senior citizen can often be kept alive if enough medical equipment and manpower are allocated to the task. Hard questions arise when the life that is thus painfully and expensively preserved is at or near the vegetable level. Little wonder that there is increasing public discussion of euthanasia, much more of it to date in Britain than in the United States. One reason may be that the economic consequences of unbridled humanitarianism—of the determination to keep people alive as long as possible regardless of cost or of the value of the lives preserved—are more apparent in a socialized than in a private medical system. Certainly British policymakers know that every penny spent on maintaining an eighty-year-old with respirators and the like is a penny that cannot be spent on the health care of the young and of those in productive age groups. And in this country there are hospitals where the doctors and nurses complain about the large proportion of beds occupied by old people who will never recover. In these hospitals it is very difficult to get beds for younger people whose chances of recovery are excellent and who still have energy and talents to contribute to society.

Aside from the degenerative diseases of old age, the most stubborn and widespread problems facing modern medicine are in the psychiatric area. Millions are disabled to a greater or lesser extent by neuroses, psychoses, drug addiction, and alcoholism and no easy solutions to these problems are evident. Yet even in this difficult area there has been significant progress. Some of the gain has taken the form of the substantially increased resources of psychiatrists, psychologists, psychiatric social workers, and other trained personnel. Even more important for the long run is the increasing understanding of how the brain works and the accompanying development of pharmaceuticals that can control or moderate many forms of psychotic behavior. Various classes of drugs are now available that can combat deep depression, curb manic overexuberance, and help restore normal or semi-normal functioning to schizophrenics. The gains should not be exaggerated, for often these drugs exact a price in creativity, vitality, and enthusiasm from those who need them. Nevertheless they have made possible a revolution in our treatment of mental illness; psychiatric hospitals can now release many more of their patients than anyone would have believed possible two decades ago. In 1960 the average daily census of the nation's psychiatric hospitals was 672,000; in 1970 that figure was down 33.5 percent to 447,000. It is an impressive achievement, though much more must be learned to help the many who need aid.

In mid-1972, when Senator Thomas Eagleton was briefly the Democratic candidate for vice-president, the nation learned the history of his past psychiatric illness and treatment. Though Senator Eagleton was forced to leave the race, it was evident that in his case psychiatric treatment had permitted him to function in public office despite his basic disability. It was an impressive example of successful psychiatric treatment.

The tragic facts about widespread drug abuse, heroin addiction, and alcoholism are too well known to require repetition here. In this area there is certainly crisis, though, curiously, there is little reference to these problems in the usual attacks on American medicine. Presumably this reflects the critics' understanding that the organization of medical care has little relevance to these scourges because we know so little medically about how to handle these behavioral pathologies. The socialized medical system of the Soviet Union has not been able to end widespread alcoholism there, and the British National Health Service has no better solution for heroin addiction than to make heroin legally available to addicts. Methadone maintenance, to date the most promising method for coping with heroin addiction, is still highly debatable and in any case represents only the substitution of one addictive drug for another. It may be that in the future chemicals will be found that can discourage or cure the tendency to employ euphoria-producing drugs. For the moment it appears that deep societal forces are responsible for these plagues and any major effort to cope with them will have to involve changes going far beyond the medical system.

Societal factors also seem to be implicated in the renewed epidemic of venereal disease, especially gonorrhea, during recent years. In the mid–1950s there was great confidence that antibiotics and public education had largely, though not entirely, extirpated the serious threats of syphilis and gonorrhea to the nation's health. In 1957, for example, there were only little more than 200,000 newly reported cases of gonorrhea. True, even then underreporting of this and other venereal diseases made the published figures unreliable, but there was general agreement that these plagues were relatively under control. By the late 1960s, however, it was unmistakable that a major epidemic was in progress. By 1969 almost 550,000 new cases of gonorrhea were reported that year, a huge rise that more than compensated for some decline in newly reported syphilis cases during the middle and late 1960s. In part this increase is related to the increasingly permissive attitudes in American society, attitudes that discourage precautions, let alone abstinence, in sexual relations. The widespread underestimation of the possible health consequences of gonorrhea is also a factor in this epidemic. Finally it is likely that the huge increase in venereal disease is in part another tragic expression of the general social pathology of the black ghettoes of the country. Here for example is the breakdown of reported cases of syphilis and gonorrhea in 1969 between whites and nonwhites in the United States exclusive of New York City.[14]

Disease	Whites	Nonwhites
Syphilis	35,078	45,736
Gonorrhea	164,419	333,759

If it is remembered that nonwhites make up little more than 10 percent of the United States population, the massive disproportion shown by these data is evident. Presumably the actual disproportion in the total population is less than indicated by these data. Private physicians probably fail to report many disease cases among their patients, while nonwhites go more frequently to clinics and other institutional providers of medical care who are more likely than private doctors to report cases of venereal disease. Nevertheless it seems likely that in venereal disease, as in drug addiction where the toll among blacks is also disproportionately high, we see another expression of the high cost of the disadvantaged position of so many of the nation's Negroes. While improved medical care in the ghettoes would certainly help, it alone would not strike at the root causes of the afflictions whose symptoms are drug addiction, venereal disease, and other illnesses born of poverty and social disorganization.

The facts reviewed in this chapter make evident that there is nothing resembling a "health crisis" in the United States. Those who speak in such terms betray their taste for fantasy and hyperbole and their ignorance of the enormous progress that has been made. Insofar as medical science can control illness and death, the United States in the 1970s has a population enjoying the best health and greatest longevity in the nation's history. To improve health and longevity further the primary need is for more knowledge to cure presently incurable diseases, for individual life styles and life patterns that will prevent the self-inflicted injuries and deaths that are now so prevalent, and for radical improvement in the material conditions of the most deprived groups of Americans.

NOTES

1. *New York Times,* December 19, 1970.
2. *Journal of the American Medical Association,* November 15, 1971, p. 961.
3. Judith R. Lave and Lester B. Lave, "Medical Care and Its Delivery: An Economic Appraisal," *Law and Contemporary Problems,* Spring, 1970, p. 256.
4. Source: National Center for Health Statistics.
5. *Leading Components of Upturn in Mortality for Men, United States —1952–1967,* National Center for Health Statistics, Series 20, Number 11, September 1971.
6. Source: National Center for Health Statistics.
7. *Ibid.,* and *Statistical Abstract of the United States 1971.*
8. *Vestnik Statistiki,* No. 11, 1971, p. 90.
9. *Demographic Yearbook 1969,* p. 579.
10. United States data from *Monthly Vital Statistics Report,* September 21, 1971. Soviet data from *Narodnoye Khozyaistvo SSSR v 1969 g.,* p. 31.
11. 1960 data from the report of the Carnegie Commission on Higher Education, "Higher Education and the Nation's Health," New York: McGraw-Hill, 1970, pp. 16–17. 1970 data from United Nations Statistical Papers, *Population and Vital Statistics Report,* based on data available as of July 1, 1971, Series A Volume 23, Number 13, *passim.*
12. *Morbidity and Mortality,* annual supplement, summary 1969 Volume 18, Number 54, p. 4 and *Ibid.,* January 7, 1972, Volume 20, Number 52, p. 1.
13. W.S. Woytinsky and E.S. Woytinsky, *World Population and Production.* New York: The Twentieth Century Fund, 1953, p. 202; *Monthly Vital Statistics Report,* September 21, 1971, p. 18.
14. *Morbidity and Mortality,* annual supplement, summary 1969, *op. cit.,* pp. 4, 14, and 62–63.

CHAPTER III

THE "DOCTOR SHORTAGE"

On a research trip to a West Coast city in November 1971, I decided to visit a physician there even though I had no appointment. Knowing that he is a first class, board-certified internist and a graduate of a highly regarded medical school, I assumed his office would be crowded and I doubted that he would have even five minutes to speak to me on my research for this book.

To my astonishment, however, the reception area was empty except for a nurse. I told her my business; she went back to speak to the doctor and then ushered me into his office. We spoke about medical economics for an hour and during that time the phone did not ring even once. When I departed, the office was as empty of patients as it had been when I arrived. The visit had occurred in midafternoon of a working day. I had seen tangible evidence that, for one doctor at least, there was a patient shortage.

Was my experience unique? Had I, by blind chance, visited the one physician in America who was not swamped with patients that day? It seems unlikely, and there is other evidence that a good deal of excess capacity exists in the American medical system. Dr. W. P. Longmire, for example,

wrote in the *American Journal of Surgery* in 1965 that
". . . in each community in our country there are a few surgeons who are doing all or more than they humanly can do.
Many, though, are working at a pace far below their capacity and this is a tremendous waste of highly skilled talent."
Dr. Longmire's conclusion is supported by a National Bureau of Economic Research study of a group of general surgeons in a suburban New York community. The study
found that a quarter of the surgeons did half of the surgical
work in the community. Even more telling is the finding
that half the surgeons studied performed on the average
each week the equivalent of less than 3.1 hernia operations,
relatively simple procedures whose execution, along with
the accompanying preoperative and postoperative care of
patients, could occupy the individuals involved only a small
fraction of a normal work week. The study concluded, "It
appears there is underutilization of valuable medical skills
in this population of general surgeons." [1]

Most public discussion of the supply of physicians ig-
nores the possibility of physician surplus and focuses instead on the "doctor shortage." Newspaper and magazine
commentators retail accounts of families moving into a
community being turned down by physician after physician
when the family sought to get medical aid. Stories are told
of seriously ill people being unable to get a physician even
when their lives were at stake. We are reminded that there
are entire communities and whole counties in this country
that do not have a single doctor resident within their bor-
ders. In recent years those spreading these chilling accounts
have frequently assured their audience that the country needs
50,000 doctors. That figure has remained constant since
the mid-1960s, though what factual base, if any, lies behind it is extremely obscure.

Let us turn to the facts now. In 1969, the Public Health Service reports, there were about 840 million physician visits in this country outside of hospitals. Assuming only that patients in hospitals saw a physician at least once a day during their hospital stay, we get roughly an additional 250 million physician visits to hospitalized patients. Adding the two we get a total of at least 1.1 billion patient-physician contacts during 1969, or an average of more than five physician contacts per United States resident in 1969. Moreover the Public Health Service statistics indicate that 54.4 percent of the population had seen a physician during the six months prior to being interviewed by a government enumerator and that 69.4 percent of the population had seen a physician during the year prior to the interview.[2]

These statistics should dispel the idea that most Americans have no access to physicians. The data also show what an enormous number of patient-physician contacts take place in the United States each year. Moreover, a large but indeterminable fraction of the roughly 30 percent of the population who saw no doctor avoided such a meeting because they felt no need to consult a physician.

But what about the supply of doctors? Has that remained static or grown more slowly than the population? The data on page 62 show that the number of physicians has grown rapidly in recent years, increasing at roughly three times the rate of population growth since the mid-1960s.[3]

These data help give new perspective to the talk about a 50,000 doctor shortage. Let us suppose that there was such a deficit in the mid-1960s when that pseudostatistic began to be used. By the end of 1971 the number of physicians had already increased by more than 50,000, yet the talk about a shortage of 50,000 still went on as though nothing had happened. Obviously such statistical myths die hard.

Year	Total M.D.'s	Total Population	M.D.'s per 100,000 Population	Population Per One Physician
1950	219,997	156,472,000	141	711
1960	260,484	185,370,000	141	712
1965	292,088	199,278,000	147	682
1970	334,028	209,539,000	159	627
1971*	345,000	211,200,000	163	612
1972**	356,000	212,700,000	167	600

* Preliminary   ** Estimate by author

Even when the United States has 100,000 more doctors than in 1965—as it certainly will later in the 1970s—some commentators will probably still be talking about the "shortage of 50,000 doctors."

By the standards of at least the past half century, this country has increased its physician supply with remarkable speed since 1960. Will the increase continue in the years ahead? To answer that question, we must look at the sources of the increased physician supply. These are basically two: the increased output of American medical schools and the increasing flow of foreign-trained physicians, including some American citizens trained in foreign medical schools, to this country.

Let us look at the rapid growth in medical schools and medical school enrollments shown by the data on page 63.[4]

Just between 1965 and 1971, the number of entering medical school freshmen rose about 40 percent while total medical school enrollment increased about a third. This reflected the progress made during the past decade in creating new medical schools and in expanding the enrollment of existing schools. The opening of additional schools in the next few years, together with the further expansion of exist-

Year	No. of Schools	Freshmen	Total Enrollment	Graduates
1950–51	79	7,177	26,186	6,135
1960–61	86	8,298	30,288	6,994
1965–66	88	8,759	32,835	7,574
1970–71	103	11,348	40,487	8,974
1971–72	108	12,361	43,399	9,500 *
1972–73	113*	13,500*	46,000*	10,000*

* Estimated.

ing institutions, it is now estimated, will permit about 15,-000 freshmen to be accepted in American medical schools in September 1975. Meanwhile the nation is now at the threshold of an even more rapid increase in the number of new M.D.'s graduated annually. In many parts of the country medical schools are reducing their required period of study from four years to three years. Simultaneously, with the most publicized lead coming from the University of Miami, the new flexibility in medical school curricula is beginning to permit Ph.D's in biology, biochemistry, and other scientific fields to enter medical school and receive M.D. degrees in periods as short as eighteen months to two years. As a result, it is not unreasonable to expect that 50,000 M.D.'s, and perhaps more, will be graduated during 1971–1975. For comparison, we may note that about 40,000 M.D.'s were graduated during 1966–1970, and 36,000 during the preceding five years.

Public concern about the doctor shortage played an important role in stimulating the remarkable expansion of American medical schools this past decade and in inducing federal and state legislatures to appropriate the money to create new medical schools and to expand existing institutions. In the private sector, medical schools benefited from public largesse as well as from private donations. All this was done in a period when many medical schools were in severe financial difficulty, more than a few of them near bankruptcy. Without public concern about a lack of physicians, it seems probable, some medical schools might have been permitted to go out of existence.

Foreign-educated doctors are the second component of this country's rapidly increasing physician supply. Their admission to medical practice here in increasing numbers offers further refutation of the idea that artificial limitations have been or are being imposed on the availability of doctors in the United States. At the end of 1963 there were 30,925 graduates of foreign medical schools (excluding Canadian medical school graduates) in this country, or about 11 percent of all M.D.'s in the United States. Eight years later the number of foreign-trained physicians here had more than doubled, reaching 62,214 or 18 percent of the total. In each of the years 1967, 1968, and 1970 more than 3,000 foreign physicians migrated to this country as permanent immigrants. In 1970 an additional 5,365 physicians came as exchange visitors or temporary workers. Past experience suggests that many of the latter will change their status to permanent residents and eventually will become United States citizens. At the end of 1971, 17,515—almost one-third—of the 52,840 interns and residents in the United States were graduates of foreign medical schools.

There are at least three major reasons for this influx of foreign physicians. One is the economic advantage of being a physician in the United States compared to being a physician in Britain or Iran or India. Additionally many foreigners are attracted to this country by the opportunity to learn the high standard of medicine practiced here. Many foreign doctors come here initially intending to stay only a few years until they have received the requisite training. Once here, however, they often marry American spouses and become accustomed to American standards of medical practice. Many despair of being able to use in their home countries the complex medical technology they have learned here, so they decide to stay. Finally, some physicians have come from Britain and some other countries because they dislike working in socialized medical systems and prefer the greater independence doctors enjoy in the United States. But even these powerful motivations would not have permitted the recent great influx of foreign physicians if United States immigration laws had not been liberalized in the 1960s to facilitate their migration and work here. Moreover, this substantial inflow would not have taken place if the American Medical Association and other concerned organizations had not welcomed these newcomers and acted to facilitate their integration into the American medical scene. There has been no attempt to hold back the foreign tide by setting unreasonably high standards for either internship and residency positions or for full licensure to practice medicine.

On the contrary, there is frequent criticism that the standards have been set too leniently, particularly as regards speaking and understanding English. Some hospitalized patients have been horrified to discover that communication with a non-American intern or resident was extremely difficult. But the great majority of foreign interns and residents working in this country have passed two screening tests: the medical and the English language examinations of the Educational Council for Foreign Medical Graduates (ECFMG). These doctors can be presumed to have at least minimum competence or better in both these areas. It would be unrealistic, however, to ignore the likelihood that a significant fraction of those who pass the ECFMG examinations are nevertheless less well qualified than the bulk of the graduates of United States and Canadian medical schools, with respect to both medical knowledge and ability to communicate in English. The resulting problems are particularly severe in those states where the great preponderance of interns and residents are foreign medical graduates. In New Jersey in 1970, for example, about 80 percent of all interns and residents were foreign medical graduates. In California that same year, on the other hand, more than 90 percent of all interns and residents were graduates of United States or Canadian medical schools. It is plain that California's climatic and other advantages were far more attractive to young American physicians than were the conditions surrounding employment in New Jersey's chief cities, Newark, Jersey City, and Trenton. It should be stressed, however, that foreign medical graduates must pass the same examinations to receive licenses as fullfledged physicians as graduates of United States schools.

The United States is not the only country that employs large numbers of foreign-born or foreign-educated physicians. One recent estimate puts the world total of doctors migrating from one country to another annually as high as 100,000. In each recipient country, the question of the quality of immigrant physicians is often raised. In this country observation at hospitals and elsewhere soon shows that some of these immigrants are superb physicians, but by no means can that be said of all. Test results give some idea of the situation.

Slightly over 66 percent of those taking ECFMG examinations ultimately obtain a qualifying certificate, but on any single examination only 35 to 40 percent receive a passing grade. Thus, many candidates repeat the test several times; currently 45 percent of candidates have taken the examination and failed on one or more previous occasions. . . . Even after they have passed the ECFMG examination and have completed requisite internships or residencies, FMG's have difficulty passing licensure examinations. Over a 35-year period the average failure rate has been 39.4 percent.[5]

These statistics suggest that the ECFMG and state licensure examinations do protect the public against receiving care from doctors who lack at least minimum qualifications. But sometimes public pressure for more doctors puts these standards in jeopardy. For example, parents of American-born students who graduated from foreign medical schools have been campaigning to lift the ECFMG requirement from these United States citizens and they have scored some legislative successes. One reason for this pressure is the unimpressive record of these United States-born foreign medical graduates when they take the ECFMG and state licensure examinations. On the other hand there are also able students among these Americans studying abroad and a new program is now making it easier for the best of them to transfer to United States medical schools with advanced standing.

The argument is sometimes made that it is immoral for the United States to depend upon foreign physicians who are badly needed in their countries of origin. A look at the data facilitates examination of this issue. The figures on page 68—supplied by the AMA—show the eight countries which, at the end of 1971, accounted for almost half of all foreign-educated doctors in the United States.

The Cuban case is the simplest since most Cuban physicians here are political refugees who fled Castro's rule. To a lesser extent, political refugees who fled from Hitler and Mussolini account for many of the Italian-educated and West German-educated doctors here. The United Kingdom

Country of Education	Number of Physicians
Philippines	7,975
India	5,081
West Germany	3,487
Italy	3,311
Cuba	2,838
United Kingdom	2,665
Switzerland	2,540
South Korea	2,353

is itself one of the world's main importers of Asian and African medical manpower, so there can be little moral objection to giving British citizens jobs here. Over half of the Swiss-educated doctors in the United States are native Americans. In the Philippines, a recent study reports, there are "approximately 28,000 physicians [of whom] ½ are in practice, mostly in Manila and other major cities, ¼ are working in the United States, and the other ¼ are not practicing at all." [6] This leaves India and South Korea as the countries to which the moral argument may apply. But there is another side to the moral argument which deserves attention.

The United States has a long and honorable tradition of having open doors for foreigners who wish to come here to improve their lives; there is no good reason why an exception to that tradition should be made against foreign physicians. Moreover, the number of foreign doctors from any country who are working here is usually only a small fraction of the physicians in the nation of origin. Even the return home of all doctors from, say, Iran or Egypt would hardly solve the medical problems of those countries, problems which in any case are born more of poverty than of physician shortage. Additionally, the right to emigrate is a fundamental human right and is so declared in a United Nations document. The denial of that right in the case of Soviet Jews, for example, has drawn wide condemnation and justly so. Why should it be heinous for foreign doctors to immigrate if there is no objection to the immigration of their fellow countrymen who are engineers or scientists or writers? Most Americans today are the descendants of immigrants who came here seeking liberty and better economic opportunity, precisely the motives impelling many of the physicians who have immigrated here this past decade.

President Nixon's 1972 Manpower Report to Congress estimated that by 1980 there will be 440,000 physicians in the United States. This estimate assumed both a continued increase in the number of medical school graduates in this country and a continuation of net immigration of foreign physicians. The report put the expected number of United States medical school graduates in 1979–1980 at 50 percent above the 1970–1971 level, i.e., well over 14,000 in absolute terms. Since population growth in this country has been slowing significantly—especially because of a sharp decline in the birth rate in the early 1970s—this estimate implies that the number of physicians will rise at a much more rapid rate than the population during the 1970s.[7] It may well be that in 1980 the United States will have about 235 million people and 440,000 physicians for a ratio of almost 190 doctors per 100,000 population, well above the present level. This could easily produce bitter complaints of a "doctor surplus," especially if there is no radical change in the present organization and financing of American medicine. Even before 1980, therefore, it is conceivable that there might be pressure to limit the surplus by restricting the immigration of foreign physicians and/or tightening the requirements they must now meet to work here as interns and residents. In effect American physicians might demand the same kind of government protection against foreign competition that is demanded today by many American industries, including steel, textiles, and shoes.[8]

Whether or not there will be a surplus of physicians in the future, the present reality is one of continuing public clamor about doctor shortages. That clamor has not been perceptibly diminished by the fact that, as of mid-1972, approximately 60,000 physicians have been added to the nation's medical manpower just since 1965. What are the reasons behind this phenomenon?

Much of the answer, as we have seen, derives from the demand side of the equation: the increasing effectiveness of medical care in curing or at least alleviating many human ills, the growing availability—through Medicare, Medicaid, and various types of medical insurance—of "free" medical and hospital care that requires little or no immediate out of pocket expenditure by the recipient, and the rising affluence of the majority of Americans, which has made the physician's fee less of an obstacle to seeking his help than it ever was before. But in this chapter we wish to focus on the supply rather than the demand side of the equation.

One major source of complaints about shortage is certainly the unequal geographic distribution of physicians relative to population. Lumping together physicians with M.D. and D.O. [Doctor of Osteopathy] degrees, the United States in 1969 had on the average 163 doctors per 100,000 population. At one extreme, Washington, D.C., had 371 doctors per 100,000 population, New York, 234, and Massachusetts, 214. At the other extreme, Alaska and Mississippi each had only 78 doctors per 100,000 population. Even this spread minimizes the actual degree of geographic inequality. Physicians tend to be concentrated in urban and suburban areas, and to be less available in rural areas. Within the cities, middle and upper class neighborhoods tend to have most of the available doctors, while few physicians reside in the low income slums. At the extreme there were 134 counties in the United States in 1969 which did not have even one physician. These counties had a total population of almost 480,000 persons, about one-quarter of one percent of this country's population. The American Medical Association's researchers have put the problem this way in their valuable handbook, *The Profile of Medical Practice:* Counties outside the nation's metropolitan areas have 26.4 percent of the country's population, but only half as large a proportion of the nation's physicians. Counties in the metropolitan areas of the United States, on the other hand, include only 73.6 percent of the nation's people but have 85.6 percent of the doctors engaged in patient care. Counties with less than 10,000 inhabitants had 2.4 percent of the nation's population, but only .8 of one percent of the doctors; metropolitan areas with over 5,000,000 inhabitants had only 12.6 percent of the people but 19 percent of the physicians.

These data make it likely that every week there are individual cases of hardship resulting from unavailability of physicians in small communities and rural areas. But the problem, though real, should not be exaggerated. Given the abundance of automobiles and other means of transport in this country, Americans can and do travel significant distances to see a doctor. Moreover, in urban communities even the most physician-bereft slum is normally only a bus, streetcar, or subway ride from a physician's office or a hospital clinic.

Once it is understood that there is a disproportionate

clustering of American physicians, a new view of the "doctor shortage" emerges. This view recognizes that at one extreme some communities have more than an adequate number of physicians and that daily an appreciable percentage of physician time in these communities goes underutilized because of a "patient shortage." Yet simultaneously other communities and neighborhoods do have an actual shortage —or even complete lack—of physicians. In purely numerical terms, physician shortage, adequacy, and surplus coexist in a complex geographic pattern over the United States. Why don't the forces of the marketplace produce a more uniform redistribution of physicians, with doctors moving from areas of surplus to areas of deficit? There are many answers to this question but one seems most important: Many physicians are willing to accept reduced incomes in order to enjoy the noneconomic advantages of preferred areas and avoid the noneconomic disadvantages of undesirable areas. For example, since the advent of Medicaid, it has been perfectly possible for physicians to earn $50,000 to $100,000 a year treating patients in the ghettoes of America's great cities. Some have taken advantage of the opportunity and the number of doctors in these deprived areas has risen. But most physicians have resisted the economic lure of the ghetto out of fear of violence directed against their person. That fear is not misplaced since each year a number of physicians practicing in slum areas are murdered or injured and physicians' offices are robbed repeatedly. Remote rural areas are unattractive to most physicians on both economic and noneconomic grounds. Precisely because of their small populations, such areas are unattractive from an income point of view. Beyond this, they have no cultural institutions and few other assets to attract physicians. One young doctor who had tried practicing in a rural area and given it up put it this way: "There was nobody around for me and my wife to talk to. The local school was pretty bad and hardly the place I wanted my kids to be educated in. And I used to worry about who would take care of me if I suddenly became seriously ill."

This discussion of the uneven geographic distribution of physicians has ignored the fact that physicians are by no means all mutually interchangeable. For an open heart operation one requires a cardiac surgeon, not a psychiatrist or a pathologist. Modern medicine can do an enormous amount to help many sick people because more than ever is now known about the human organism and how to correct its malfunctions. But this volume of knowledge is too great for any one man, or even for any group of two or three men. The abundance of knowledge forces specialization and the investment of additional years of training beyond medical school to get requisite skills. In the status ladder of American medicine the specialist commands both higher fees and greater prestige than the general practitioner. Moreover, the medical schools of the United States—precisely because of their emphasis on scientific medicine and on research to increase medical knowledge—have been dominated by specialists who have been the professional career models held up to medical students as they decided their futures. Little wonder that the trend in recent decades has been for a rapid increase in specialists and even of subspecialists. The old days, for example, when a radiologist was expected to diagnose lung cancer in a chest film one minute, give X-ray therapy the next, and then perform a thyroid scan with radioactive iodine are disappearing. Instead we are getting such subspecialists as neuroradiologists and experts in nuclear medicine who confine themselves each to one small corner of what used to be the radiologist's universal domain.

Statistics tell the story of the decline of the generalists and the rise of the specialists. Let us define medical generalists to include the general practitioner, the new breed of family physicians, internists, who specialize in internal medicine but who have increasingly in recent decades taken over many of the functions of the GP, and pediatricians. In 1931, there were 117,000 generalists, or primary physicians, out of a physician total of 156,000. The generalists were 75 percent of all American doctors. In 1970 there were 118,000 generalists out of 334,000 physicians, only about 35 percent of the total. In these four decades, the population of the United States rose very sharply while the supply of primary physicians remained virtually unchanged.

Presented this starkly, the picture is overdrawn. The specialists have taken over many of the functions of the general practitioner. They perform much more of the surgery, deliver many more of the babies, set many more of the broken arms and legs, and treat many more of the nation's neuroses and psychoses than they did in 1931. Except in isolated areas today's primary physician limits himself to a much smaller fraction of all possible medical interventions than he did four decades ago. Moreover, the statistics are somewhat misleading because they ignore the fact that many who are technically specialists also act to some extent as primary physicians. The psychiatry or pathology resident who "moonlights" by working in a hospital emergency room or making house calls for neighborhood physicians taking a weekend off are familiar features of today's medical scene. So is the surgeon who lets his neighbors know he will be glad to look at their everyday aches and pains because his surgical workload is too small to occupy all his time. There seem to be no comprehensive statistics on the matter, but much fragmentary evidence suggests that each year a great deal of primary medical care is delivered by individuals who are classified as specialists in the data on physician manpower.

Nevertheless, there can be little doubt that much of the public complaint of "doctor shortage" is really complaint about "primary physician shortage." Useful as anesthesiologists, neurosurgeons, pediatric urologists, otolaryngologists, ophthalmologists, allergists and their fellow specialists are, they are not what the average American family wants when it is looking for a doctor to minister to father's influenza or baby's diarrhea. The volume of public complaint suggests strongly that there are many communities with inadequate numbers of primary physicians, though again there are undoubtedly other communities in which no such shortage is felt.

Data reported in the *AMA Newsletter* for August 14, 1972, shed some light on the imbalance between supply of and demand for different types of physicians. In 1971 that organization's physician placement service had more than twice as many calls for general practitioners as it had registrants for such posts. But conversely the number of surgeons seeking places was five times as great as the number of opportunities, while the placement service had only one pathology opening for every ten pathologists who applied.

Such evidence suggests that there are too many physicians in particular specialties, for example, general surgery and neurosurgery, while the nation could use more primary physicians and also more specialists in other fields, for example, ophthalmology and dermatology. Again we have the problem of why physicians do not leave overcrowded fields for areas of greater need. Some do, of course, but hardly in adequate numbers. In part this reluctance to change is motivated by the additional years of training required to shift, say, from neurosurgery to dermatology after the individual in question has already made a large investment of time in acquiring his first specialty. The need for additional education is minimal for the specialist thinking of becoming a primary physician, but to many doctors the prospect of becoming a primary physician is uninviting because the job is seen as uninteresting. "Why should I spend 80 percent of my time with hypochondriacs, colds, and upset stomachs?" one young surgeon snorted when asked about turning to general practice. And one psychiatry resident who had been a general practitioner explained he had left his lucrative practice as a primary physician because "I was really doing psychiatry most of the time without any training so I decided I might as well get the training and be a real psychiatrist."

Correcting the current maldistribution of physicians —both geographically and in terms of specialization— will not be easy. We have already referred to some of the non-economic factors involved, but there are economic forces at work as well. The available data show that there are significant differences in the net earnings of physicians depending upon their specialties and on where they work. In *The Profile of Medical Practice,* American Medical Association researchers have reported that in 1969 the average surgeon in a metropolitan area enjoyed a net income of $49,260, more than twice the $24,643 earned by a psychiatrist in a non-metropolitan area. General practitioners, on the other hand, did economically better in non-metropolitan than in metropolitan areas, averaging $38,782 in the former locations and $32,689 in the latter.

If we lump all types of physicians together and look at the regional variation throughout the country, we find the highest 1969 average net earnings to have been received in the East South Central states where the average reached was $45,704 in metropolitan areas. The lowest average net earnings was received by physicians in the non-metropolitan areas of New England where the average was $31,379. It is interesting that overall the lowest net earnings in the United States in 1969 were received by physicians in New England and the Middle Atlantic states, in many parts of which physician competition is very keen because of the relative abundance of doctors in, for example, the New York, Boston and Philadelphia metropolitan areas. Presumably many physicians feel the economic disadvantages of New England and the Middle Atlantic states are compensated by the cultural advantages, the abundance of well-equipped hospitals and major medical centers, and other non-economic factors.

Some have urged saturating the medical system, i.e., turning out so many physicians that the sheer force of competition and economic necessity will finally provide a doctor for every small town and ghetto street in the country. But nobody seems to have calculated the number of physicians this country would need to make this solution work. And there are warnings from other countries that sheer numbers of physicians do not solve the problem. We have already noted that in the Philippines a quarter of all graduate doctors do not practice though there is a great shortage in rural areas. The experience of the Soviet Union and the Eastern European countries also reveals that even when a nation graduates very large numbers of doctors, it is still hard to staff undesirable areas and some doctors prefer to abandon their profession rather than work in the boon-docks. But there is an even more serious objection to this "solution": the medical version of Parkinson's Law. Sharply increased competition among physicians would create the tendency to overtreat, overprescribe, and overoperate. The critics already charge that unnecessary operations are performed in this country simply because some doctors want to augment their income. The excessive number of tonsillectomies performed in this country gives some support to this view, though the issue is more debatable on other procedures. But any serious effort to flood the American medical system with doctors is likely to increase the incidence of overdoctoring of all kinds, to the detriment of many patients.

A second suggestion involves the use of compulsion, in effect making all doctors subject to a non-military draft. The government, it is held, should intervene and tell physicians where to practice and in what fields of medicine. In effect this would amount to conscripting the nation's physicians and forcibly redistributing them according to some bureaucrat's idea of where they ought to work and what kind of work they should be doing. The constitutionality of such drastic measures is open to doubt; the immediate impact of such a scheme would be to make medicine a much less desirable field both for existing practitioners and for young people thinking of a medical career. Moreover, a doctor working under the threat of going to jail is likely to be resentful and to show his bitterness in his work. In any case, the problem of redistributing physicians is hardly so urgent that it justifies depriving physicians of the basic freedoms all other Americans enjoy.

Both of these types of "solution" deserve to be rejected. Instead there is every reason to suppose that a whole variety of measures, tailored to fill the needs of different communities and different situations, can meet much of the present problem where it exists, without unreasonable cost or unfair and self-defeating compulsion. Let us look at five approaches:

1. The Emergency Health Personnel Act of 1970 authorizes the Secretary of Health, Education, and Welfare to send doctors, dentists, nurses, and other health workers into scarcity areas at the request of local health agencies and with the approval of local governments and medical societies. This legislation is still in early stages of implementation and only a few communities are being aided, but it has possibilities. This approach certainly deserves stronger support than is provided by the relatively small sums so far appropriated for it. Many young physicians today proudly call themselves health activists and proclaim their undoubtedly sincere aim of helping the poor and the unserved sick. They form a potential reservoir of medical manpower whose recruitment could implement this legislation on a much wider scale than has taken place to date.

2. In some areas, for example, Santa Clara County, California, there have been successful experiments with what has been called "the doctor's second office." This is an approach toward easing the local maldistribution of physicians; that is, communities which are well supplied or even oversupplied with physicians may be near other communities suffering severe shortages or having no doctors at all. A medical society or other agency may alleviate this situation by setting up suites of physicians' offices in the scarcity region and arranging to have them manned in rotation by doctors from the areas of plenty. A variation of this idea that is being used in some states is the practice of creating mobile medical units which are staffed with requisite per-

sonnel and travel regularly to different towns or neighborhoods that lack their own physicians and nurses. These ex-
pedients also deserve expanded use.

3. In many parts of the country, hospital outpatient
clinics and emergency rooms have become increasingly significant sources of outpatient medical care, particularly at
night and on weekends and holidays. The number of outpatient visits in community hospitals almost doubled from
70,727,000 in 1962 to 133,545,000 in 1970 and the
growth has continued in 1971 and early 1972. Many hospitals are now going into the business of providing ambulatory medical care for non-emergency patients. They are
building appropriate outpatient facilities and hiring experienced physicians to staff them, rather than relying primarily on interns and residents. As this is written many hospitals are considering forming Health Maintenance
Organizations to offer comprehensive prepaid medical and
hospital care to groups residing in the neighborhoods
served by these hospitals. With adequate financing, such institutions as Harlem Hospital in Manhattan's famous Negro
district and Lincoln Hospital in the Puerto Rican and
Negro ghetto of the East Bronx could become major centers for providing health care to the deprived populations
they serve. Moreover, in these and other violence-plagued
areas, it is probably more realistic to expect that doctors
and nurses will be willing to work in a hospital environment where adequate security measures are possible than in
traditional solo practice offices which are so vulnerable to
the desperate narcotics addict turned robber or mugger to
get the money he needs to buy heroin.

4. There are many measures the community of doctors
is taking and others it might take. The American Medical
Association has encouraged the development of a specialty

of family practice, whose new entrants receive advanced training so they can provide better primary care than was possible for the less well trained general practitioner. The medical profession needs to take a hard look at specialty training with a view to modifying the number of training opportunities in the light of society's needs for different types of practitioners. Any such examination would undoubtedly disclose that there are opportunities to reduce the flow of future specialists into already crowded fields and to increase that flow into specialties where significant shortages are being felt. A complete moratorium on the entry of new trainees might be declared for a year or two or three in the most overcrowded specialties, while government subsidy might be sought to provide financial incentives for younger specialists in surplus fields to enter training residencies in deficit specialties.

It is particularly heartening that medical schools have begun to put more emphasis upon primary medical care, bringing general practitioners and family physicians into the classrooms and using them as field preceptors with whom medical students may work to get a taste of what everyday primary medical practice is like. A separate problem is the need to provide the residents of many communities over the nation with physician coverage for emergencies every day of the year and twenty-four hours of every day. This problem has already been solved in some communities through cooperative arrangements among local physicians or through special medical organizations set up to provide weekend, holiday, night, and vacation coverage for physicians requesting it. But it is inexcusable that there are communities where such arrangements do not exist, and where a patient calling his doctor outside of office hours sometimes finds his physician unavailable and no substitute provided. The medical profession has a positive obligation to assure that patients can get their own physicians or suitable surrogates at all times. And while more physicians make house calls than popular legend admits, the widespread discontent on this issue suggests more should be done to provide physician or nurse visits at home to patients who really require them. On the other hand it must be noted that many patients ask for house calls which are not medically essential. Many other people move into a community and make no advance contacts with a physician before they are ill, then become outraged because a doctor who does not know them refuses to make a house call in response to a 2 or 3 A.M. telephone request. There are mutual obligations in the patient-physician relationship rather than, as too many people seem to think, all obligation being the physician's.

5. There has been much discussion about the desirability of introducing a new type of health worker termed variously a physician's assistant, a physician's associate, and a MEDEX. These persons are trained for relatively short periods and then employed by doctors to assist and, to some extent, to substitute for them. A small number of these persons have already been trained and are working and there are plans to expand their numbers.

No doubt such ancillary personnel can be helpful, but some caution about any all-out effort to expand their numbers seems advisable. In many cases nurses who have received additional training—nurse-practitioners, pediatric nurses, operating room nurses—are already performing many of the duties now envisaged as suitable for physician's assistants. It would seem more sensible to upgrade the training and responsibility of nurses—an established category of health workers—than to rush pell mell into training many thousands of physician's assistants. Nurses are understandably resentful that physician's assistants, who have trained for shorter periods and have less knowledge than many nurses, are being paid higher salaries.

Certainly experimental employment of physician's assistants is worthwhile, but before this country decides to train large numbers of them, a hard look should be taken at the whole field of medical personnel so that an integrated policy can be adopted. The alternative a decade from now could be the existence of three hostile groups, physicians, physician's assistants, and nurses, with the physician's assistants seeking more of the prerogatives of physicians and the nurses assailing both the other groups as male "sexists" blocking women nurses who want to climb the rungs of the medical career ladder. The nation's pool of medical workers is already plagued by a number of bitter quarrels between groups seeking to defend their prerogatives and others seeking to expand their jurisdictions. A prime example in some states recently has been the angry struggle between physicians and nurses over the efforts of the nurses to gain what medical societies assert are the privileges of practicing medicine. The need now is for more flexibility in the use of available trained men and women, not for the injection of a new large and distinct interest group that could further complicate an already difficult and delicate situation.

It should not be ignored that some spokesmen for the black community have already denounced the idea of physician's assistants as part of a plot to provide only "second class people and second class care" for the poor and deprived. These charges are probably unjustified, but they reflect the feeling many people have that when they feel sick they want to see a full-fledged doctor and not some less well trained substitute. It is a sentiment that cannot be ignored.

In any case, the outlook is for a rapid increase in the

number of physicians of all kinds in the years immediately ahead. This increase is unlikely to solve all problems people have in mind when they complain about "doctor shortage," but it should help ease many of them. In this connection, it also seems relevant to recall that only a few years ago there was great national alarm about the shortage of chemists, physicists and other scientists with Ph.D. degrees. Now many in the expanded number of Ph.D. scientists recently graduated find that they are a glut on the market and have difficulty finding jobs. There would seem to be a lesson here for those who make exaggerated claims about the "doctor shortage" and want a great and rapid increase in the number of M.D. graduates.

The constant drumbeat of complaints about shortages in the American medical system is so great that many readers may be surprised that there is at least one major area of surplus. The United States has too many hospital beds, in large part because of earlier overenthusiastic efforts to remedy the "hospital bed shortage." In 1971 probably more than $4 billion was expended on maintenance of empty hospital beds. Those who see the solution of the nation's medical problems in grandiose new programs to increase every type of medical manpower and facility would do well to ponder the implications of the hospital bed surplus.

We are indebted to the American Hospital Association sample survey of short-term general and special hospitals —roughly, community hospitals—for the basic facts. In 1971 these hospitals had on the average 836,397 beds but for the entire year the occupancy rate was only 75.9 percent. On the average, in other words, almost one out of four community hospital beds stood empty during 1971, the equivalent of about 200,000 empty beds. Since this is a national average, the situation was better in some areas and worse in others. In December 1971, when the national occupancy rate was below 70 percent, only 63.4 percent of all beds in the Pacific Coast states were occupied, i.e., more than one out of every three beds in California, Oregon, and Washington was empty. In New England, the area with the highest rate that month, only 75.9 percent of the available beds were occupied.[9]

An American Hospital Association estimate has put the cost of maintaining an unoccupied bed at the two-thirds the cost of maintaining a bed occupied by a patient. In 1970, the 186,560 hospital beds vacant on an average day cost about $10 million daily, or about $3.6 billion for all of 1970. Since there were about 200,000 empty beds on the average day in 1971 and since hospital costs were greater in 1971 than in 1970, the hospital bed surplus must have cost $4 billion or more in 1971.

A House Ways and Means Committee report gives some essential background on how this situation arose:

> Bed capacity of community hospitals totaled 826,000 in 1969—75 percent above the 1946 level. In terms of beds per 1,000 population, community hospital beds have increased from 3.4 to 4.1 since 1946. Trends in output also have shown considerable growth: Admissions and patient days per 1,000 population increased 44 and 33 percent, respectively, both greater than the increase in bed capacity.
>
> The growth essentially reflects the implementation of programs to resolve the need for acute-care beds. The Hill-Burton program, which began in 1947, was largely responsible for bed capacity expansion. As of December 31, 1970, the program had provided Federal funds for the construction of some 336,000 beds.[10]

Until 1970 the nation's hospital occupancy rate had been increasing each year since World War II, reaching a peak of

78.8 percent in 1969. But in 1970, the rate fell to 78 percent and the preliminary indication, as noted above, is that the rate declined to 75.9 percent in 1971. The number of people admitted increased slightly in 1971 to 30,260,125, a gain of .4 percent. But the average length of stay declined 1.3 percent and the total number of inpatient days declined 1.5 percent. The most notable decline was 3.2 percent in the average length of stay of patients 65 and over, mostly Medicare patients.

In 1970 and early 1971 some hospitals began to suffer from lack of business and were forced, in some areas, to reduce their staffs. This unexpected development was blamed on the recession and its accompanying unemployment. But, although the recession and unemployment were not notably worse in 1971 than they had been in 1970, the drop in occupancy rate accelerated. Those who had believed that the 1970 decline was the result of lapsed health insurance policies had to take another look. Perhaps the pressure to cut medical costs by discouraging physicians from hospitalizing patients and urging them to get patients out of the hospital as soon as possible was beginning to be felt. Moreover, the nation's birth rate was dropping precipitously, making hospital obstetrical wards disaster areas from the financial point of view.

An animated national discussion began in mid–1971 as to what should be done with the unneeded hospital facilities. The California Medical Association, for example, commented: "Various short-range alternatives exist for hospitals, and, to a certain extent, for geographic areas where hospital occupancy rates are especially low. These include closing down inefficient institutions, temporarily closing down specific sections within individual hospitals, coordination of services among various hospitals within an area, and converting facilities from one use to another." [11] At the American Hospital Association convention in Chicago in mid-1971 high government officials suggested such alternatives as leasing unneeded hospital areas to entrepreneurs conducting other businesses, or converting surplus hospital capacity to playgrounds for employees' children or to methadone clinics for heroin addicts.

The decline in occupancy rate may be a temporary phenomenon; many hospital administrators devoutly hope so. But whether temporary or permanent the financial distress and loss caused by this surplus capacity was a useful reminder that the United States can have surplus medical capacity.

NOTES

1. E.F.X. Hughes, V.R. Fuchs, J.E. Jacoby, and E.M. Lewit, "Surgical Workloads in a Community Practice." New York: National Bureau of Economic Research, 1971.
2. Data on nonhospital physician visits are from the Public Health Service publication, *Current Estimates from the Health Interview Survey United States—1969,* p. 3. Hospital visits by physicians estimated from American Hospital Association data.
3. American Medical Association, *Reference Data on Socioeconomic Issues of Health 1972,* p. 41.
4. Sources: *Journal of the American Medical Association,* November 22, 1971 and information from the Association of American Medical Colleges. Estimates prepared by author.
5. Thomas D. Dublin, "The Migration of Physicians to the United States," *New England Journal of Medicine,* April 20, 1972, pp. 873–874.
6. *Ibid.,* p. 875.
7. *American Medical News,* May 1, 1972.
8. Much of the preceding discussion is based on data in the medical licensure and education issues of the *Journal of the American Medical Association,* June 14, 1971 and November 22, 1971 respectively, the AMA's *Foreign Medical Graduates in the United States,* Chicago, 1971, and the 1972 edition of *The Profile of Medical Practice.*
9. "Hospital Indicators," *Hospitals,* March 16, 1972, p. 19.
10. *Basic Facts on the Health Industry.* Prepared for the use of the Committee on Ways and Means by the staff of the Committee on Ways and Means. Washington: Government Printing Office, 1971, p. 46.
11. "Declining Hospital Occupancy Rates—Temporary Problem or Impending Crisis?" *Socio-Economic Report,* California Medical Association, April 1972, p. 5.

CHAPTER IV

THE END OF THE MEDICAL
COST EXPLOSION

In preceding chapters we have argued that several popular stereotypes are wrong. We have pointed out that the statistics do not support a doomsday vision of a national health crisis. We have also maintained that since the United States now has more physicians than ever before in its history, the usual complaints about a "doctor shortage" are exaggerated and the real problem is more one of geographic and specialty maldistribution. Now we must point out that the notion of a medical cost explosion is obsolete, at least for the present. The total cost of medical care did increase sharply from 1965 to mid-1971 as a result of both rapidly rising medical prices and increased utilization. But beginning in August 1971, President Nixon's new economic policy drastically slowed the inflation in hospital charges and doctors' fees. Between August 1971 and August 1972, the medical price index rose only 2.2 percent, substantially less than the cost of living rise in the same period.

The data below supply the basic facts about the growth of United States expenditures for medical care and related purposes since the late 1920s: [1]

Fiscal Year Expenditures

	1928/29	*1949/50*	*1965/66*	*1970/71*
	(*billion dollars*)			
Total	3.6	12.0*	42.1	75.0
Public expenditures	.5	3.1	10.8	28.5
Private expenditures	3.1	9.0	31.3	46.5
Direct payments	2.9	7.1	18.9	24.2

* Total affected by rounding.

The main elements of this picture are plain enough. Between the late 1920s and the beginning of the 1970s, expenditures related to medical care climbed almost 21–fold. Government spending in this field rocketed in 1970/71 to 57 times the 1928/29 level. Private spending rose relatively less and was only fifteen times the 1928/29 level in 1970/71. One component of private expenditures, direct payments by consumers, increased least and was only eight times as high in 1970/71 as in 1928/29.

Another important point emerges from these data: The tendency for United States medical-related expenditures to rise rapidly is not new. In the mid–1960s, this country spent about 3.5 times as much in this area as it had in 1950. The long term upward trend in medical expenditures reflects most fundamentally the growth of the nation's population, the increase of its wealth, and the high priority put on health and medical care. And the trend is international, for medical care expenditures have risen rapidly in many other advanced industrial countries, not just in the United States.

Here, for example, is the description of the situation in Sweden that appeared recently in the Blue Cross magazine *Perspective:*

Inflation in Sweden's health cost has been extraordinary: in one period, per capita cost of health care increased by 164 percent compared with an increase in the U.S. of 174 percent. Sweden's rate of increase in health costs has "slowed" to only 14 percent per year, compared with a U.S. rate of 10.4 percent; but, even at the "new" rate of increase, a situation could be produced in which Sweden—by 1987—would be spending 37 percent of its GNP on health, compared with the current U.S. rate of 7 percent. Of course, necessity will dictate that something be done . . . but even the most hopeful government official sees Sweden spending no less than 13 percent of its national income on health in that year.

In the United States there was substantial acceleration of the rate of increase of health care expenditures after the mid-1960s. Between 1965/66 and 1970/71 health-related spending for the nation as a whole jumped roughly 80 percent. The chief item in this rapid inflation was government expenditures, which nearly tripled. The smallest increase took place in direct payments by consumers, which rose somewhat less than 30 percent. Intermediate was the increase in private insurance payments for health expenditures, which rose roughly at the same rate as total spending.

Medicare—the federal government program for paying hospital and doctor bills for persons 65 and over—and Medicaid—the combined federal-state program for financing medical care of the poor and near-poor—are the new factors which made the difference. In 1965/66 federal, state, and local governments disbursed about $1.8 billion for health insurance for the aged and for medical payments under public assistance. In 1970/71 these two categories —Medicare plus Medicaid—accounted for expenditures of almost $14.5 billion. This amount was more than the nation's entire medical spending in 1950. The costs of both programs have far exceeded original estimates and innumerable cries of anguish have been heard from angry Congressmen and Senators who have had the unpleasant job of facing the fiscal and tax consequences of these added strains on an already overburdened national budget. At the state and local levels, too, the ballooning costs of Medicaid have produced consternation and vigorous efforts to try to contain them.

But the impact of Medicare and Medicaid has been substantially greater than is suggested by the dollar amounts spent directly on these programs. Medicare and Medicaid have given major impetus to the general inflation in medical care prices. The whole history is a classic example of what happens when government acts without really understanding what it is doing, or what the impact of its actions will be. Congress enacted these programs in the mid–1960s without really weighing the consequences; it made no serious effort to increase resources for medical care although it had legislated an increased effective demand. The result was entirely predictable. The sudden infusion of billions of dollars of new purchasing power into a medical market place with a relatively fixed supply of resources—at least in the short run—promptly pushed prices up for almost every element in the health care system. Since politicians dislike admitting their mistakes, scapegoats had to be found on whom to blame the medical cost inflation. Soon the press and other media were denouncing the "greedy" doctors and the "grossly inefficient" hospitals. It apparently could not be admitted that what was happening was an entirely predictable example of the working of supply and demand in a free market. To make the medical price inflation worse than it might have been, Medicare and Medicaid took effect just when the United States was rapidly boosting its spending on the Vietnam war, which further fanned the inflation in the economy as a whole. Thus medical cost inflation was superimposed upon general inflation. The effect on hospital charges and physicians' fees is shown below: [2]

| Fiscal Year | Hospital Daily Service Charges | | Physicians' Fees | |
	Annual Index (1967 = 100)	Percentage Increase Over Preceding Year	Annual Index (1967 = 100)	Percentage Increase Over Preceding Year
1967	92.2	16.6	96.9	7.4
1968	106.4	15.4	102.8	6.1
1969	120.5	13.3	109.1	6.1
1970	135.4	12.4	117.0	7.2
1971	152.8	12.9	125.8	7.5

The increases in hospital charges and physicians' fees have certainly been substantial this past half decade. But do they represent profiteering or immoral behavior or heedless greed, as so many critics assert? It is hard to see how hospitals can be charged with profiteering since the great majority are nonprofit institutions. No owners draw dividends from Massachusetts General Hospital in Boston or Presbyterian and Bellevue Hospitals in New York City.

One major factor behind the increases in hospital charges is the rising cost of labor in this labor-intensive industry. According to American Hospital Association data, the average payroll, or labor, cost per patient day almost doubled between 1965 and 1970. In 1965 the labor cost was $16.70 per patient day; in 1970 it was $33.16. Part of this jump represented an increased number of workers, a 20 percent rise in hospital personnel between 1965 and 1970. All or most of the remainder of the increased labor cost must have reflected climbing wage rates. Since a large fraction of hospital workers—orderlies, laundry workers, cleaning personnel, nurses' aides, etc.—have historically been among the lowest paid laborers in American society, it is precisely these most impoverished workers who have been among the chief beneficiaries of these wage increases. The sudden torrent of Medicare and Medicaid funds made it financially possible for hospitals to raise wages for their lowest paid workers to more nearly decent and adequate levels. Inevitably many of the beneficiaries were blacks, Puerto Ricans, Chicanoes. Are we to term these disadvantaged workers profiteers?

In some areas unions have led the struggle of the poorest hospital workers to get decent wages. Speaking in November 1970, the president of New York City's Drug and Hospital Union Local 1199 noted that in 1960 hospital wages in New York were so low that 20 percent of these workers were on welfare. In 1970, by contrast, none was on welfare. Wage increases during the decade had raised the lowest hospital pay from $27.50 a week in 1960 to $110 a week in 1970, with a further increase in minimum pay to $130 scheduled to go into effect in July 1971.[3] A Bureau of Labor Statistics study found that New York City hospital workers on the average increased their wages by 30 percent between 1966 and 1969, about twice the rate of increase in wages for factory workers. General duty nurses in New York City had lower wages than factory workers in mid–1960 but by March 1969 their earnings had increased to a level one-third greater than that of factory workers. Similar dramatic hospital wage increases took place all over the United States. Here is how the Bureau of Labor Statistics explained the background of this national trend:

The major increase in daily hospital charges, especially since 1966, reflects the rapid demand rise for hospital services, the consequent need to attract new workers to this field, the use of more expensive equipment, and significant gains, many of a catch-up nature. The latter factor is of particular significance in hospitals which are both traditionally low-paying compared to other industries and labor-intensive in that payrolls account for more than three-fifths of hospital expenses.[4]

Professor Martin S. Feldstein has suggested that there may also have been a philanthropic element in the steep wage rises of hospital workers in recent years. He writes: "A hospital, as a philanthropic or public organization, may concern itself with the welfare of its staff as well as of its patients. The tradition of low pay for hospital staff developed when hospital budgets were very tight and the institutions were largely dependent on voluntary philanthropic support. More recently, the rapid rise in the demand for hospital care has given hospital administrators much greater freedom in determining salary levels." The administrators, Professor Feldstein believes, raised wages above those required by strictly market conditions, presumably defending this policy by the need to pay "decent" salaries in order to improve the quality of their work force, raise morale, reduce turnover, etc.[5]

A second factor is evident in hospital cost and price increases. Because they were being paid by the government and by insurance companies on a cost reimbursement basis, hospitals had a strong incentive to buy and install new, more complex, and more expensive equipment developed as part of modern medical technology. All over the country in recent years there have appeared intensive care units, heart-lung machines, kidney dialysis units, and the like. The ability of hospitals to help save lives has increased but so has the cost. Put most simply, the life-saving and curative potentials of a hospital stay are now much greater than they were in the early 1960s because the average hospital is better equipped than it used to be. The higher price now for a day's hospital stay is, on the average, payment for a better product, but this consideration is usually ignored in denunciations of the rapid rise in hospital costs.

In the most modern hospital intensive care units, for example, each bed is equipped with heart monitors, pumps, ventilators, automatic blood and urine analyzers, cardiac pacemakers, computer-controlled infusion systems and other equipment whose use requires a one to one nurse-patient ratio. A ten-patient unit needs additionally three respiratory therapists, one mechanical technician, one electronic technician, a physician, a nursing instructor, and a ward clerk for each eight hour shift around the clock. And these are not the most expensive installations. Renal special care units and other very specialized life-saving installations can cost more than $400 a day. More moderately priced but hardly cheap is the special unit for badly burned patients at the University of Michigan hospital in Ann Arbor, which can handle as many as 160 patients at a cost of up to $215 a day for each.

These remarks are not intended as a blanket justification for the increases in hospital costs and prices since the mid–1960s. The permissive atmosphere of the early Medicare days, when there seemed to be no limits to cost reimbursement, must have encouraged slack habits and wasteful practices. In some communities there was needless duplication of expensive equipment—cobalt bombs for radiation therapy are a favorite example, as are heart-lung machines for open heart operations in hospitals where such procedures might be done only once a week or even less often. Undoubtedly the present pressures on hospitals to cut costs or to slow their growth are useful. But we should beware of expecting too much efficiency from hospitals. Taking care of sick people—especially sick elderly people, who now comprise a large fraction of the average hospital's patient load—is a very expensive matter, requiring large amounts of labor and much complex equipment. Care cannot be mechanized like the production of paper clips or tin cans. If it is to be humane, it cannot be an assembly-line operation on the model of automobile factories.

There is every reason to expect that future technical and medical advances will permit still more impressive feats of life saving but at still higher costs, since even more complex machinery and a higher worker-patient ratio will be required. It is staggering, for example, to think of the costs if the immunological problems that have so far discouraged heart transplants were suddenly to be solved so that such transplants became frequent, routine operations.

What about physicians? As we saw earlier, their fees have gone up substantially since the mid–1960s, though at a rate only half that of hospital charges. Those who argue that physicians are profiteering usually justify their conclusion by comparing the rise in physician fees with the increase in the Consumer Price Index. But there are tens of millions of Americans whose wages have increased more rapidly than the cost of living in recent years. Are they all profiteers? Some union leaders have been among the most vociferous critics of higher medical costs, including physicians' fees. In their own negotiations for their members, these union leaders never seem to regard a wage increase limited to the cost of living as acceptable.

Between 1967 and December 1971 the Consumer Price Index rose 23.1 percent, while the index of physicians' fees rose 32.2 percent. The difference is appreciable. But its significance is reduced if we recall that in this same period physicians' costs for such items as office rent, wages of nurses and other physicians' aides, and malpractice insurance rose steeply. Moreover, the constant increase in medical knowledge and its rapid application for patient care means that each year the average physician can do more to help the average patient than he could the year before. There is no allowance for this productivity or quality improvement in the mechanical comparison of physicians' fees over time.

Does it really make sense to compare physicians' fees only with the Consumer Price Index? Physicians' fees are payment for work done. They are labor incomes like the wages and salaries earned by persons in other occupations. Once this is realized, a more meaningful series of comparisons can be made: [6]

	1965	1970
	(1967 = 100)	
Physicians' fees	88.3	121.4
Compensation per man hour, total private economy	88.4	123.6
Building trades workers union minimum hourly rate	90.9	128.8
Printing trades workers union minimum hourly rate	93.0	121.2
Truck drivers and helpers union minimum hourly rate	91.2	122.5
Local transit operators union minimum hourly rate	89.8	125.2

Physicians' fees have risen sharply but so have most other earnings in the American economy since the mid-1960s. Physicians' fees, these data show, actually increased slightly less rapidly between 1965 and 1970 than average hourly compensation in the total private economy of this country. They rose more slowly than hourly earnings of construction workers and local transit workers, and slightly more rapidly than wages of printers and truck drivers. Other data show that physicians' fees rose less during 1967–1970 than salaries of policemen and firemen and one had only to read the newspapers during 1969–1971 to learn of many union contracts providing annual wage increases of 10 to 15 percent. These gains were substantially higher than the corresponding annual percentage increases in physicians' fees.

None of this conflicts with the fact that physicians, on the average, earn substantial incomes. But those incomes are in part the product of a relatively long work week, 51.3 hours a week on the average in 1969 according to an American Medical Association survey. Physicians' incomes of $30,000 to $50,000 a year reflect the high degree of skill, knowledge, and responsibility expected of them, as well as compensation for low incomes or no income at all during the lengthy period of training after high school. There are physicians who earn extraordinarily high incomes, far above the average. These are usually men with special skill and knowledge and such individuals always command superior earnings in any field. When a Muhammed Ali and a Joe Frazier can command millions of dollars for a single fight and a Ralph Nader can charge $2,500 for a single hour-long speech, it is not surprising that some outstanding physicians can and do earn annual incomes in excess of $100,000.

All elements of the medical care community have entered a radically new economic climate since President Nixon imposed price and wage controls in the summer of 1971. The government is clearly dismayed by what it regards as the runaway inflation of health care costs. Having unleashed this inflation by introducing Medicare and Medicaid into an unprepared medical economy in 1966, the government now seeks to deal with the consequences by imposing upon individual health care professionals the strictest controls placed upon any element of the American economy.

Even before the price and wage freeze in mid-1971, it was apparent that both federal and state governments were determined to cut medical care costs in any way possible. Major political battles took place in California, New York, and other states which attempted to cut the level of benefits for Medicaid patients. In the case of both Medicaid and Medicare, serious efforts were begun in the late 1960s to tighten up on claims by scrutinizing them more severely and by trying to cut payments wherever possible. In mid-1970, for example, the agencies responsible for screening and paying physicians' Medicare claims were reducing about one-third of them, with the average claim being cut 7.3 percent. By the first quarter of 1971, almost half of all physicians' Medicare claims were being cut, with the average reduction per claim about 11.5 percent.[7] In the early days of Medicare only 3–4 percent of physicians' claims had been reduced. Beginning in 1969, moreover, the Bureau of Health Insurance of the Social Security Administration began placing ceilings on physicians' fees. First, in 1969, it put this ceiling in each area at the 83rd percentile of comparable fees paid doctors in 1968. At the beginning of 1970, the authorities announced that they would now permit the use of customary 1969 fees, rather than 1968 fees, as the basis for physician reimbursement but they moved the ceiling down from the 83rd percentile to the 75th percentile of fees charged in each area. Then in July 1971 the ceiling was placed at the 75th percentile of customary 1970 fees in each area. Meanwhile, well before the price freeze was announced in mid-1971, Congress was trying to limit increases in prevailing fee levels to a percentage tied to the cost of professional practice and to income levels in the economy as a whole. Faced by these added controls, the American Medical Association began acting like a labor union. In January 1970 it issued a public protest at the setting of Medicare fee ceilings without opportunity for preliminary comment. It argued that the action amounted to paying Medicare doctors in 1970 on the basis of a ceiling reflecting 1968 fees, despite rapid inflation elsewhere in the economy and despite physicians' higher costs.[8]

By the beginning of 1970 the trend toward controls on physicians' fees was clearly visible. This undoubtedly prompted physicians to raise their rates as much as they could. Fee increases in fiscal years 1970 and 1971 both averaged over 7 percent annually compared with the 6.1 percent increases in the two preceding years. There was nothing surprising in this behavior. People generally try to protect their own interests in the light of the trends they see operating. Perhaps the main surprise is that the fiscal year 1970 and 1971 fee increases were little more than in earlier years despite the growing likelihood of government controls.

Physicians' fees were not the only element of medical costs under pressure in the late 1960s and early 1970s. The government moved to curtail payment for use of nursing homes, to reduce hospital admissions, and also to cut the length of patient stays in hospitals. Perhaps as a result of this pressure, average length of stay in community hospitals, which had risen from 7.8 days in 1965 to 8.4 days in 1968, declined to 8.3 days in 1969 and 8.2 days in 1970. In 1971, the average length of stay for Medicare patients

—i.e. persons sixty-five and older—in community hospitals was significantly below the 1970 level. But for non-Medicare patients, i.e., persons under sixty-five, the average length of community hospital stay was roughly the same as it had been in 1970.[9]

These and other efforts to restrain cost increases by limiting fees and curbing utilization were not without effect. In fiscal year 1971 the nation's health care expenditures rose 10.7 percent, a substantial increase but still the smallest annual percentage rise since the adoption of Medicare and Medicaid. This slowdown took place despite a 25 percent increase in Medicaid expenditures. That rise presumably reflected the impact of the recession in making more people —the increased numbers of the totally or partially unemployed—eligible for Medicaid benefits. In the case of Medicare, payments to doctors during fiscal year 1971 increased only slightly, while there was a decline in payments to nursing homes. These signs of successful restraint appeared despite the fact that the number of people eligible for Medicare increased during fiscal 1971.[10]

President Nixon's August 1971 price and wage freeze and its sequel, the Phase II period of control, profoundly affected the medical care economy. The effectiveness of the President's program in slowing the pace of medical price inflation became quickly apparent. Between 1966 and 1970, the average annual increase of the medical care component of the Consumer Price Index was about 6.5 percent. Between December 1970 and December 1971, however, that component rose only 4.8 percent, i.e., substantially less rapidly than the average of the preceding four years. This was no mean achievement, especially if it is remembered that the freeze was announced after more than half of 1971 had already passed into history. By mid-1972 the inflation in medical care prices had become history. Between August 1971 and August 1972, the medical care component of the Consumer Price Index increased only 2.2 percent, well under the 2.9 percent rise in the total CPI for the same twelve months. Yet, ironically, much public debate at that time continued to ignore this historic change.

The sudden slowdown in medical cost and price inflation in the second half of 1971 is so important that it is worth looking at in more detail. The overall impact is best seen by comparing the annual percentage increases in the relevant components of the Consumer Price Index beginning with December 1966: [11]

	12 months ending December				
	1967	1968	1969	1970	1971
	(annual percentage increases)				
Consumer Price Index	3.0	4.7	6.1	5.5	3.4
CPI medical care index	6.4	6.2	6.0	7.3	4.8
Physicians' fees	6.1	5.8	7.3	8.1	5.2
Dentists' fees	5.1	5.1	7.5	5.5	6.4
Hospital daily service charges	15.4	13.3	12.0	13.5	8.9
Drugs and prescriptions	−.2	.4	1.1	2.5	1.3

The sudden dramatic nature of the change caused by the President's price freeze is best realized if we look at the quarterly behavior of these indexes of medical care costs during 1971. (See page 104.)

As the data below show, the medical care component of the Consumer Price Index was actually less in December 1971 than it had been in September 1971. This reflected the adjustment made in October each year to include changes in the price of health insurance which is not shown

| | 3 months ending | | | |
| | March | June | Sept. | Dec. |
	(percentage changes)			
Consumer Price Index	.6	1.4	.6	.7
CPI medical care index	2.1	1.4	1.4	− .2
Physicians' fees	1.8	1.5	1.2	.5
Dentists' fees	2.1	1.3	1.4	1.4
Hospital daily service charges	3.4	2.2	2.4	.7
Drugs and prescriptions	.7	.8	0	− .1

separately as a component of the medical care figure. Perhaps the most dramatic statistic in the above is the December 1971 quarterly increase in hospital service charges, .7 percent. This was the lowest quarterly rate of increase for this item since the quarter ending in June 1962, almost a decade earlier. These data also contain an unsolved mystery: Why did dentists' fees rise as rapidly in the December quarter—when the freeze was the dominating element—as they had in the previous quarter? And while the physicians' fee index for the last quarter of 1971 increased much less than it had in any of the previous three quarters, more detailed data show that there were increases of well over 1 percent during that quarter for office visits to pediatricians and psychiatrists as well as for hernia repair operations. These curious exceptions to the general deceleration of medical care costs in the last months of 1971 suggest that enforcement difficulties may arise if the effort to control prices by government fiat is continued for very long.

By mid-1972, it was indisputable that President Nixon's price control program had stopped the medical cost explosion. In earlier years following the inauguration of Medicare and Medicaid, the rise in health care costs each month and each year had frequently been the largest of any major component in the Consumer Price Index. As of this writing, however, the medical field has lost that undesirable distinction, and health care prices are actually rising less rapidly than the overall cost of living index.

The change has been very dramatic and very quick. During 1967–1970, we have seen, the annual increase in the Consumer Price Index medical care component varied from 6.0 to 7.3 percent. In 1971, the imposition of price and wage controls in August helped cut the medical care price increase between December 1970 and December 1971 to 4.8 percent. In mid-1972 the Bureau of Labor Statistics released data showing that medical care prices had risen only 2.6 percent between July 1971 and July 1972, an increase less than the corresponding 3.0 percent increase in the overall Consumer Price Index. In that same period the rise in housing prices had been 4.0 percent and in food prices 3.7 percent, both significantly higher than the medical price increase.[12] Some observers began to question whether this successful containment of medical price rises might not ease the pressure for radical restructuring of the medical care system. Much of that pressure, as noted earlier, had its roots in anger at the rapidly rising costs of medical care after Medicare and Medicaid were introduced.

Let us now look more closely at the price control mechanism by which medical cost inflation was contained after mid–August 1971.

For the health care field, the price freeze theoretically lasted four months, rather than three months as for most of the rest of the economy. It was not until mid–December 1971 that Price Commission regulations defined permissible increases in prices and charges for medical care. Part of the delay was presumably due to the fact that the Price Commission waited to be guided by the conclusions of the special 21-member Advisory Committee on the Health Services Industry. This committee included representatives of both providers and consumers, with the latter holding the upper hand. The controls were severe and were applied differentially to institutional and noninstitutional providers. Noninstitutional providers—physicians, dentists, medical laboratories, Christian Science practitioners, midwives, blood banks, birth control clinics, etc.—were limited at most to aggregate price increases of 2.5 percent over the levels of November 14, 1971. Even these increases were permitted only to reflect allowable cost rises. Institutional providers, primarily hospitals and nursing homes, were treated more gently. They were permitted to raise prices up to 6 percent without prior permission. Any price increases beyond 2.5 percent had to be registered with local price enforcement authorities, who also had to receive justifications of these increases. Any institutional provider wishing to increase prices more than 6 percent had to request formal advance permission, with the request being screened first by newly established State Advisory Boards.[13]

The harshness of the price controls imposed upon health care professionals was underlined by the nature of the appeals procedure: a physician, dentist, or other health professional wishing to raise his fees beyond 2.5 percent had to request specific permission from the Internal Revenue Service director in his district. His appeal had to show why he wanted an exceptionally large increase, i.e., more than 2.5 percent, demonstrate "serious hardship or gross inequity," and make clear that his appeal was "not part of a plan" to avoid the purposes of the price and wage control legislation. The difference in standards being applied to different groups was illustrated by the Pay Board's decision in January 1972 to cut back from 12 to 8 percent the increase won by aerospace workers—members of the United Automobile Workers—in contract negotiations. The UAW filed suit in February 1972 to have the Pay Board decision set aside because that body had allegedly acted in a "discriminatory, arbitrary, illogical, and capricious" manner. The suit also contended that the aerospace workers had been denied the due process required by the price control law because the board failed to hold public hearings or to provide transcripts of caucuses. Leonard Woodcock, president of the union, was vociferous in defending the right of his members to a 12 percent wage increase; apparently he had no quarrel with the 2.5 percent limit placed on health professionals. As a leading advocate of Senator Edward Kennedy's national health insurance proposal, Mr. Woodcock had often denounced the soaring cost of medical care but he saw nothing wrong with the soaring wages of his members. In March 1972 Mr. Woodcock and three other labor leaders resigned from the Pay Board when the pay raise of about 20 percent won by the West Coast longshoremen after a long strike was reduced to 15 percent—six times the percentage rise permitted for doctors' fees.

To many physicians, dentists, and other individual providers of health care services, the regulations governing them seemed grossly discriminatory and unfair. They noted that no other professional field was subject to such draconian rules and they were irked, too, by the stringent limitations on appeals. It did not escape their attention that the Pay Board established a 5.5 percent increase in wages as automatically acceptable, while simultaneously granting much larger increases to strong unions of coal miners, construction workers, railroad workers, etc. The California Medical Association spoke out sharply, accusing the Price Commission of "discriminatory, unjust, and unrealistic" restrictions on physicians. Individual California physicians competing with the Kaiser-Permanente groups had a special reason for bitterness. The solo practitioners were limited to a 2.5 percent increase in fees; the Price Commission permitted the Northern California Kaiser-Permanente medical organization to raise premiums to its million subscribers by 10.32 percent.

In effect the 2.5 percent ceiling set for physicians and dentists represented a political judgment in Washington which included at least two elements: (a) a feeling that millions of Americans were angry at what they considered excessively high medical costs and would welcome a severe crackdown in this field, and (b) a conviction that physicians and dentists could not and would not strike and therefore had no effective way to protest. Apparently physicians were so indignant over these new controls that they began to badger the American Medical Association to act like a union and exert "doctor power." At any rate the AMA felt it necessary to explain to its members why it could not be a union. Here is how the AMA weekly, *American Medical News,* put the matter editorially in its issue of January 31, 1972:

> The American Medical Association is not a trade union, nor, under present conditions, can it become one. . . . When [a labor union] negotiates for wages, it's called collective bargaining and that's legal.
> However, physicians who are not compensated on a salary basis but who derive their income on a fee for service, capitation, or any other basis from the public are independent contractors. If they negotiate as a group for payment, it's called price fixing and that's illegal.

In this and other ways, the AMA was trying to discourage physician militancy, while seeking to present an image of cooperation in the national price control effort. The AMA leaders were aware that their organization and its members had a public relations problem. But the AMA does not control the nation's doctors. Even before price controls, it was being assailed by a portion of its physician constituency as too liberal and too weak in its actions to defend doctors' interests. Certainly any national policy under which doctors, dentists, and others felt they were being severely discriminated against would tend to encourage their militant elements to find ways to evade the existing regulations, to try to have the regulations changed, or, if all else failed, to defy the law. There could be trouble ahead in this field, trouble implied by the recent growth of unions of doctors.

It was noted earlier that much of the current debate about altering the American medical system has arisen from concern about costs. Not only has the absolute volume of spending risen sharply, but so also has the percentage of gross national product devoted to these purposes. The latter rise has also been a long term phenomenon. In fiscal 1950, national health expenditures were 4.6 percent of the GNP; in fiscal 1965 the percentage had risen to 5.9 and in fiscal 1970 and 1971 the corresponding percentages were 7.1 and 7.4. The last two figures probably exaggerate the trends, however, because the recession of the early 1970s slowed the rise of the national income. A year of vigorous economic recovery which also saw continued effective control of rising medical care prices might well witness some decline in the percentage of the GNP devoted to national health expenditures.

In the first half of 1971, at the request of the House Ways and Means Committee, the Department of Health, Education, and Welfare prepared estimates of national health expenditures in fiscal year 1974. These estimates were prepared first on the assumption that there was no legislative action affecting the medical system in this country and then on the assumption that various of the bills before Congress were passed and put fully into effect by fiscal 1974. Because of the timing involved, the estimation process took no account of the price and wage freeze announced in mid–1971. Nevertheless, the estimates and assumptions underlying them are worth considering for the light they may throw on the future of medical costs and expenditures.

In the table below, actual national health expenditures in 1971 fiscal year are compared with the HEW estimate for fiscal 1974 on the assumption that no major legislative change will have taken place by then. When the 1974 estimate was calculated, the 1971 data given below were not yet available. In addition, the 1974 estimate was made before the institution of price and wage controls in mid–1971.[14]

	1971 Actual	*1974 Estimate*
	(billions of dollars)	
Total health expenditures	75.0	105.4
Hospital care	29.6	43.9
Professional services	20.4	27.9
Drugs and appliances	9.4	11.6
All other	15.6	22.0

Essentially, HEW estimates that without any change in existing legislation national health expenditures in fiscal 1974 will be 40 percent higher than in fiscal 1971. For this to be realized, national health expenditures would have to increase an average of more than 11 percent annually during fiscal 1972–fiscal 1974. This possibility cannot be ruled out, but the passage of time since the estimate was prepared during the first half of 1971 has made such an outcome less likely. We now know that the percentage rise in fiscal 1971 national health expenditures was less than during any earlier year since the mid–1960s, indicating a deceleration in earlier inflationary trends. Moreover in fiscal 1972 the rate of increase of medical prices and costs has slowed dramatically, while pressures to restrict utilization are continuing. It would require a new intensification of medical cost and price inflationary trends between mid–1972 and mid–1974 to turn the $105.4 billion fiscal 1974 estimate into reality. As this is written that estimate looks too high, and, assuming no major new health legislation is passed over this period, a fiscal 1974 figure of $95–$100 billion seems more reasonable. An even lower total is conceivable.

The reason the assumption that no major new health legislation is passed is so central is because all of the health insurance bills before Congress in the early 1970s would have the effect of raising medical expenditures. In one way or another, they would tend to narrow still more the area of direct payment, while increasing the area in which government or private insurance would pay for health care services. The marginal cost of additional health services would thus seem zero, or at least cheaper than full price, to additional millions of potential patients. In the HEW study referred to above, the "induced cost"—i.e., the additional cost resulting from higher utilization when a type of medical care is made to seem "free"—assumed to exist for various services was as follows:

> Hospital care—25%
> Extended care facilities—25%
> Physician services—25%
> Dentist services—45%
> All other professional services—35%
> Drugs—35%
> Eyeglasses and hearing aids—40%

The authors of the HEW study note that these are rough estimates based on a review of the scanty available statistical
evidence. They also note that if it were not for limitations
of supply the percentage of induced cost for institutional
care and physician services might be even higher than the
estimates given above.[15] One can debate whether these estimates of induced cost are too high or too low but certainly
the phenomenon itself must be taken into account in calculating costs of proposed legislation. For some of the more
ambitious health insurance bills considered by the 92nd
Congress, the HEW estimates that induced costs might vary
from $6.9 billion to $11.3 billion. The three most expensive health insurance programs before Congress, it was estimated, would put national health expenditures at
$113–$115 billion in fiscal 1974.

As noted earlier, all elements of this theoretical analysis
have been outmoded by developments in the year since it
was made. The imposition of price and wage controls on
almost the entire economy has raised new perspectives and
so has the trend toward tighter utilization controls in the
medical system. Yet passage of a comprehensive national
health insurance bill would inevitably arouse great expectations and stimulate demand for all types of health care services substantially. In the atmosphere of new, greater shortage of personnel and facilities thus created, it would be
more difficult than ever to maintain price controls over
health care providers. On the contrary, there would be
the danger of unleashing a new inflation of health care
prices and costs such as was initiated by Medicare and
Medicaid in 1966.

NOTES

1. *Social Security Bulletin,* December 1971, p. 11.
2. *Ibid.,* p. 21.
3. *New York Times,* November 25, 1970.
4. *Ibid.,* June 5, 1970.
5. Martin S. Feldstein, "The Rising Cost of Hospital Care," Washington: Information Resources Press, 1971, p. 68.
6. *Statistical Abstract of the United States, 1971,* pp. 62, 224, and 226.
7. *Medical Economics,* September 13, 1971, p. 213.
8. "HEW Methods in Changing Medicare Law Questioned," AMA news release January 11, 1970.
9. Data from the American Hospital Association in *Hospitals,* August 1, 1971, p. 462 and March 16, 1972, p. 17.
10. *New York Times,* January 18, 1972.
11. This table and the one that follows it are taken from a memorandum by Loucele A. Horowitz of the Division of Health Insurance Studies of the Social Security Administration.
12. *New York Times,* August 22, 1972.
13. The full text of the order appears in *New York Times,* December 16, 1971.
14. Dorothy P. Rice and Barbara S. Cooper, "National Health Expenditures, 1929–71," *Social Security Bulletin,* January 1972, p. 7 and *Analysis of Health Insurance Proposals Introduced in the 92d Congress.* Washington: U.S. Government Printing Office, 1971, p. 128.
15. *Analysis . . . , op. cit.,* p. 83.

PAYING FOR
MEDICAL CARE

We turn now to consider how medical care costs are paid for
in the United States and who pays them. These are important matters because different modes and sources of payment profoundly affect the behavior both of patients and of
those who care for them. Most people tend to be economi-
cal, careful and calculating about expenditures from their
own pockets. They know that they are surrendering alternative goods and services in order to buy the goods and services they do acquire. Conversely the incentives to economy and prudence tend to be least where individuals do not
see that they are making sacrifices when they use some
scarce resource, but believe instead that they are receiving
"free" goods or services. These considerations are particularly important in the medical field because, as we have
seen, so much of present medical care in this country is
seen to be "free" by its recipients, while there is intense political agitation to make all medical care "free."

The abuse of the environment provides a useful case in
point. Until recently there seemed to be no costs involved
in polluting the air, the seas and the earth itself. In effect it
was generally believed that the environment provided a

"free" receptacle for all gaseous, liquid, and solid wastes generated by human activity. Now, of course, opinion has shifted sharply, and it is widely understood that the thoughtless disposal of waste products actually carries very high costs in environmental deterioration. The result has been a proliferation of government and other regulations aimed at reducing pollution, while there have been many suggestions for imposing taxes and other costs on those who defile the air and water around us all. It has all been a classic example of the abuse of "free" resources. The implicit lesson emerging from this sobering experience has many applications elsewhere, not least with regard to the many proposals for making health care "free."

Contemporary methods of paying for medical care in this country can be classified in several different ways. The most useful distinction is between direct payment by the person (or some close relative) who receives the service and third party payment by some seemingly distant source. In this country the third party payers are typically private insurance companies (including Blue Cross and Blue Shield) or some agency of government under a variety of programs that range from those of the armed forces and the Veterans Administration to Medicare and Medicaid. Other agencies of government provide, finance, or supervise such other third party sources of medical care payment as workmen's compensation, maternal and child health programs, school health programs, and various experimental efforts at health care delivery to the poor under the direction of the Office of Economic Opportunity and the Department of Health, Education, and Welfare. In the past, an appreciable amount of medical care was delivered free of charge to the recipient either because physicians donated their services or because philanthropic individuals and groups paid the costs involved. Today, however, the role of private philanthropy in paying for medical care (about 1.5 percent of national health expenditures) is so small that it can be safely ignored here. Medicare and Medicaid reduced the need for physicians to donate their services, but they did not eliminate this philanthropy. Some physicians work without pay, for example, in the free clinics which have sprung up in various communities to serve "street people" and other special groups. And even under Medicaid some physicians prefer to treat indigent patients without charge rather than cope with the paperwork involved in getting Medicaid payment.

A generation ago, in fiscal 1950, direct payments accounted for more than two-thirds of all personal health care expenditures, 68.3 percent to be exact. Even in fiscal 1965, just before Medicare and Medicaid became law, direct payments provided more than half—52.5 percent—of personal medical expenditures. In fiscal 1971, that percentage was down to only slightly more than one-third of the nation's personal health care expenditures, 37.2 percent. The massive shift from direct to third party payment was not enough, as we have seen earlier, to prevent the money amount of direct payments from increasing. The sums involved rose from $7.1 billion in fiscal 1950 to $24.2 billion in fiscal 1971. But measured as a percentage of gross national product, direct payments remained remarkably stable at slightly less than 2.5 percent of GNP in calendar years 1950 and 1970. The sharp increase in total national medical expenditures as a percentage of GNP over these two decades was entirely accounted for by the explosive growth of third party payments.

The virtues of direct payment as a means of cost control can only be envied by those charged with the formidable problems of cost containment for third party payers. The

typical consumer who has to pay for medical care out of
his own pocket thinks twice or even more often about seeking that care and he has an incentive to shop around to
learn what the prices of alternative physicians, hospitals,
etc. will cost him. It is interesting that a prominent reformer
among state insurance commissioners, Dr. Herbert Denen-
berg of Pennsylvania, has recently placed much stress upon
consumers knowing the alternative prices charged in different hospitals in each area of that state. That information is
relevant for the man or woman who must pay his own bill;
it can hardly seem terribly relevant to the individual who
knows his hospital costs, whatever they may be, will be
paid by an insurance company or a government agency.
The same considerations apply to the Price Commission
order in late 1971 that physicians make their fee schedules
available for patient inspection. From the physician's or
hospital's side, too, knowledge that the consumer has to pay
the bill exerts a restraining influence. In the case of physicians this knowledge was undoubtedly the origin of "Robin
Hood medicine," i.e., the policy of charging patients different fees depending upon the doctor's evaluation of what
they could afford to pay. And hospitals, in the days when
most of their bills were paid by patients, were much more
concerned with limiting costs than they became after 1965
when Medicare and Medicaid arrived.

Of course medical care is not comparable with standardized commodities like cans of soup. The consumer in
1960 who shopped for the cheapest doctor and the cheapest hospital might have been betraying his own fundamental interests by denying himself first class care, at least to
the extent that price differences among medical care providers then reflected quality differences. But if the consumer
was not terribly ill and had a self-limiting illness, say, in-

fluenza in a healthy twenty-five-year-old man or woman, any licensed doctor would be qualified to give him such limited aid as medical science could provide for his illness. On the other hand, if he or she had rapidly progressing advanced melanoma, there was little that even the best hospital or physician could do to save the patient's life. Between these two extremes is an important and large area of sickness in which the quality and qualifications of the physician and the hospital can affect the duration, severity, and outcome of illness significantly. The interplay of the variables of price, quality, and outcome of treatment in medical care is a complicated matter which is too often oversimplified.

Private medical insurance is, in terms of number of people covered, the most important form of third party payment in this country. The most popular type of insurance pays for hospital care over some period. In 1940 12.3 million Americans had hospital insurance; in 1970 181.6 million had it. Some of these insured persons were individuals over sixty-five who had coverage supplementary to Medicare. If we restrict ourselves to persons under sixty-five, 83.5 percent of Americans had hospital insurance at the end of 1970; 80.8 percent had insurance for surgery; and so on down to 48 percent who had coverage for doctors' office and home visits, 15 percent for nursing home care, and 10.3 percent for dental care.[1]

Private medical insurance is a fiercely competitive field in which many organizations are involved and many types of policies are offered. The dominant type of private health insurance is the group contract covering the labor force of a single employer or of a group of employers, a contract whose cost is increasingly paid for, entirely or in large part, by employers.

In this common situation, the pressure for economy is felt keenly by employers and by union negotiators. The employer wants to minimize the cost of the medical insurance he pays for his employees since it is an element of his production cost. The union official sees the cost of the medical package in a labor contract as an amount of money that reduces the sum the worker receives in visible, welcome money wages. But to the individual union member, his medical insurance is given; it costs him no more if he uses it to the hilt. There is no incentive for economy on his part short of the point at which his coverage is exhausted. He saves nothing, gets no rebate or other monetary reward if he does not use his medical insurance. Finally the development of major medical insurance policies has tended further to attenuate the policyholder's interest in economizing on use of medical resources, though the situation would be worse if these policies did not usually have deductibles and co-insurance provisions which force the user to bear part of the cost.

The dominance of hospital insurance and in-hospital benefits makes matters still worse. This creates the temptation to press the doctor for admission to the hospital where costs are paid as against ambulatory care where costs are usually not covered by insurance. To some, the solution seems obvious. Just extend insurance to cover ambulatory services, such as outpatient diagnostic tests. But the experience of the Federal employee health insurance program in the early 1970s showed the matter is not that simple. In that case the extension of Blue Cross-Blue Shield coverage to out of hospital diagnostic tests generated such a huge increase of demand that the insurers suffered a large loss. The cure, in this case, was apparently worse than the disease. Once out of hospital diagnostic tests were made "free," neither the insured nor their physicians had any motive to economize, with the result mentioned above. Diagnostic tests are particularly sensitive to this effect because so much of the demand for medical care comes from hypochondriacs and the functionally ill. With the wisdom of hindsight it is now apparent that for a person to go into the hospital for diagnostic tests often represents some sacrifice of convenience and perhaps even of wages. The sacrifices are less if out-of-hospital tests are "free" and the physician is then less restrained by fear of imposing too heavy a financial burden on his patient.

An increasingly popular way out of these dilemmas is greater emphasis upon utilization reviews and upon exhortations to physicians and patients alike not to abuse their insurance privileges. But exhortations are not famous for effectiveness, and even those who give them are restrained by the nightmare that the one time a patient was denied a test or a hospital admission for economy reasons might be the one time he really needed the test or the hospital admission. Even hypochondriacs eventually get sick and die and repeated demonstration of cancerphobia is no guarantee that the person involved may not some day actually develop cancer. Utilization reviews cost money and they can irritate both doctors and patients.

Nevertheless the tendency now is to tighten the utilization reviews. One possible direction for the future surfaced in Philadelphia in early 1972. There a local judge held the admitting physician responsible for hospital costs incurred by his patient, costs Blue Cross had refused to pay. In that case a physician admitted the patient to a hospital for what Blue Cross claimed were diagnostic tests, a type of admission not covered by the patient's Blue Cross contract. The judge agreed with Blue Cross and held the physician liable for the approximately $500 involved. Simultaneously but independently, Philadelphia hospitals and the city's Blue Cross organization agreed on a set of principles which included a provision that patients would not be held responsible for costs of hospital admissions Blue Cross reviewers deemed unnecessary. Pennsylvania Insurance Commissioner Herbert S. Denenberg indicated his opinion that in such cases the admitting physician would be the appropriate person liable for costs.[2]

The issue has not been finally decided as this is written. But it is worth speculating about the possible consequences of a final decision that physicians are personally liable for the costs of hospital admissions that Blue Cross reviewers deem unnecessary. Even in that situation physicians would still have to balance their fear of financial liability from such adverse decisions against the peril of being sued for malpractice by the patient and also the risk that lack of hospitalization might in some way endanger the patient. In this uncomfortable position physicians might demand that Blue Cross take the responsibility for denying hospitalization before the fact, rather than afterward. But if Blue Cross takes on the burden of prehospitalization clearance, it also makes itself the potential target of suits from doctors and patients displeased by these decisions.

There is a simpler way out of these dilemmas. Unfortunately, there is no sign yet that it is likely to be implemented soon. This simpler solution is the elimination of what is usually called front end or first dollar health insurance, i.e., insurance that pays health care costs starting with the first dollar of expense. If hospital insurance contracts were limited by law so that they could pay costs only after, say, the first few days of hospitalization, patient and doctor alike would have a greater interest in economizing on hospital use. Professors Richard N. Rosett and Robert L. Berg of the University of Rochester have criticized Blue Cross' devotion to first dollar insurance and they have recalled that Blue Cross was originally formed to help protect hospitals against uncollectible debts. Professors Rosett and Berg write:

> Conventional insurance controls, deductibles and coinsurance return to the consumer the job of monitoring and enforcing efficiency. If Blue Cross were to offer an insurance policy under which the subscriber paid for the first seven days in the hospital himself, more than half of all bed days would be paid for directly rather than through the insurance company. This would provide a powerful incentive for efficiency, but it would return the problem of bill collection to the hospitals. Blue Cross stubbornly resists this solution to the problem of soaring hospital charges.
>
> If such a deductible were adopted, it is true that some bills would be uncollectable, or collectable only at great expense, and that this expense would be passed on to the consumer, but this is true of department stores, too. Such expenses are in fact far outweighed by savings that would result from forcing the suppliers to ask themselves what the customers will be willing to pay for.[3]

A related argument has been made by Harvard Professor Martin Feldstein in his recent book, *The Rising Cost of Hospital Care*. He maintains that the effect of hospital insurance is to stimulate hospitals to make available much more expensive care than patients really want. He asserts that patients with hospital insurance ask for relatively expensive hospital care because it seems cheap or free to them at the time. Professor Feldstein writes, "This induced demand for expensive care gives a false signal to hospitals about the type of care that the public wants." But when the bill has to be paid for the excess demand thus generated, i.e., when Blue Cross and other private insurance companies have to raise their rates sharply to pay for the increased cost, the public outcry demonstrates that the community really did not want as much hospital care or as expensive care in hospitals as it actually was buying. The same reasoning, in all probability, applies also to surgery in this country. It has been shown that many operations are performed much more often, relative to population, in the United States than in Britain. That does not automatically prove that too much surgery is being performed here since the data may mean that too little surgery is being performed in Britain. Nevertheless the fact that surgical insurance is so widespread in this country raises the possibility that Americans are much more willing to undergo less essential or perhaps even needless operations than they would be if they had to pay the full cost of such procedures.

But, the reader may object, in Britain most medical care is socialized and the hospitalized patient pays directly neither for his hospital stay nor his operation. Why then are there so many fewer operations in Britain than in this country? The answer is provided by an observation in Professor Mark Pauly's book, *Medical Care at Public Expense:* "In the British National Health Service (NHS), usage of hospitals is controlled not by limits on demand but by restrictions on supply. Hospital use in the United Kingdom was greatly restrained in the postwar years because the government built almost no new hospitals. Thus the quantity of services rendered could not exceed the quantity that it was technically feasible to render, and use was held down." As we shall see later, a somewhat similar strategy of restricting costs and usage by holding down the supply of hospital beds has been applied by the Kaiser-Permanente prepaid medical groups.

Professor Herbert E. Klarman of New York University has carried this reasoning and experience one step further.

He has suggested studying the feasibility of cutting the nation's medical costs by curtailing the number of hospital beds available. He notes that research by medical economists has shown that, all other things being equal, hospital utilization in this country varies with the supply of beds.[4]

There is considerable merit in the arguments advanced by the scholars quoted above, but the political pressures in this country work in the opposite direction. All the major national health insurance schemes propounded by President Nixon, Senators Kennedy and Javits, and others aim to make expensive medical care seem more freely available than it is at present. The Nixon Administration's proposal has the relative merit of providing for deductibles and some degree of coinsurance but probably far less than needed to prevent serious further abuse of "free" care. In all this there was further evidence of the flight from the market regulation of demand and supply in medical care without adequate realization of the new difficulties that arise as the market is weakened and its regulatory functions fall more and more into the hands of bureaucrats.

The emphasis above has been on the problems that the spread of private health insurance has brought in its wake. But this insurance has also made important contributions. The wide availability of first class medical care to most Americans is in part the result of the fact that private health insurance has eased the burden of sickness, financially at least, for tens of millions of Americans. Just between fiscal 1950 and fiscal 1971, the percentage of the nation's personal health care expenditures paid through private health insurance tripled from 8.5 to 25.5 percent, while the absolute amounts paid leaped from $879 million to $16.6 billion. Health insurance payments and rates have increased so rapidly because of the rise of medical care

prices, the trend toward continued expansion of benefits offered subscribers and the tendency for insured people to
utilize medical services more than uninsured people do.

The essential policy problem for the nation is how to
balance the advantages and disadvantages of health insurance. Doctrinaire conservatives might argue for the aboli-
tion of health insurance on the ground that it encourages
waste of scarce medical resources and weakens incentives
for economy. The national decision against any such extreme individualism was made long ago, and wisely so. But
what is dismaying is that the equally extreme and doctrinaire position holding that all health care should be made
"free" commands such significant support inside and outside of Congress. Any such scheme, if adopted, will undoubtedly impose heavy needless costs because of the
waste and abuse that must inevitably arise whenever scarce
resources are declared "free." The politicians now backing
such ideas undoubtedly relish the immediate political benefits their position gives them. But if they are responsible
leaders, they must reckon also with the Pandora's Box of
troubles their schemes will impose upon society. The experience with Medicare and Medicaid has already provided
more than a little sobering knowledge of the sorts of problems likely to bedevil the nation's medical system and society as a whole if any broad and seemingly generous system of national health insurance is adopted. It is to the
operation of these programs that we now turn, therefore.

MEDICARE

Long decades of bitter political struggle reached a cli-
max in 1965 when Congress passed and President Johnson
signed into law the bill enacting Medicare and Medicaid.

The political forces that had won were jubilant, and some of the winners saw their breakthrough as the beginning of quick further progress toward a system of comprehensive national health insurance. Their dejected opponents saw the same possibilities ahead and their reaction, of course, was one of apprehension. But by the early 1970s, the attitudes of the contending forces had changed significantly. The opponents of national health insurance were pointing to the experience under Medicare and Medicaid as important arguments against rushing into a national health insurance scheme of any ambitious proportions. The proponents of national health insurance were arguing that they had learned from the mistakes committed under Medicare and Medicaid and had new proposals that would avoid similar fiscal debacles. The nation as a whole had gained some sobering lessons from these two programs, and at least some of the starry-eyed naivete of the mid–1960s had vanished under the hard pressure of experience. In this section we shall review the Medicare program, while the next section will be devoted to Medicaid, the two programs whose total cost in fiscal year 1973 President Nixon, in his January 1972 budget message, estimated at $17 billion.

Medicare, which went into effect on July 1, 1966, provided for two government-financed programs for medical care for those sixty-five and older. The Hospital Insurance (HI) component covers the full cost of hospital care for sixty days after payment of an initial deductible charge which began at forty dollars in 1966 and had risen to sixty-eight dollars by January 1972. A Medicare beneficiary is entitled to an additional thirty days of hospital care but he must pay a quarter of the deductible amount—$17 a day at present—for each of these thirty extra days beyond the initial sixty day stay. These benefits can easily amount to

$10,000 during a Medicare patient's hospital stay for ninety days, but there are more benefits available. On the 91st day of a period of extended hospitalization, the Medicare patient can begin to get help from his additional sixty days of "lifetime reserve" during which he must pay half of the deductible amount—$34 a day at present—toward his hospital bill. Of course most Medicare patients recover from a particular illness and leave the hospital before the first ninety days are up. If they remain out of the hospital for sixty days or more and get sick again thereafter and must re-enter the hospital, the entire cycle of benefits begins all over again. This can be repeated as long as a Medicare patient follows the pattern of being in the hospital for ninety days or less and then stays out of the hospital for sixty days or more thereafter.

In addition to these hospital benefits, the HI component of Medicare provides benefits for treatment in extended care facilities following hospitalization, benefits which cover full cost for twenty days and full cost minus one-eighth of the deductible for another eighty days. HI is financed by the Social Security payroll tax and the associated tax on self-employed individuals, taxes which have had to be raised repeatedly in recent years partly because of the rapidly mounting costs of Medicare. More than 95 percent of the persons sixty-five and over are covered by HI. The cost of coverage for persons who were sixty-five or older when Medicare went into effect, and thus could not contribute to it if they had retired, has been met from general tax revenues.

Additionally, Medicare includes what is at this writing a voluntary Supplementary Medical Insurance (SMI) program. This pays 80 percent of the "reasonable and customary" charges, above a fifty dollar deductible, for physicians' services, diagnostic tests on an outpatient basis, radiation therapy, etc. This is paid for by a monthly premium that began at $3 in 1966 and rose to $5.80 in July 1972.

The importance of Medicare is indicated just by the numbers of people involved. Hospital Insurance covered slightly more than 19 million people on July 1, 1966, a figure that had risen to 20.4 million four years later. The SMI enrollment is slightly lower but also includes the great bulk of Americans sixty-five and over.

The humanitarian arguments for Medicare are real and important. The aged are the most likely to be ill and frequently their sicknesses are life-threatening and very expensive to treat. Heart disease, cancer, stroke, diabetes, arthritis, and other major killers and cripplers hit hardest at the elderly. Yet at the same time most older people are retired and do not have current earnings to pay for medical care. But many of the elderly do have savings in addition to Social Security and private pensions, as well as children who are able to contribute to their parents' upkeep, including medical care if necessary.

The elderly did not go without medical care before Medicare, of course. Many paid for it then out of their own or their children's pockets; some estimates suggest that more than half had private medical insurance; and others received care without charge from the Veterans Administration, welfare programs of different governmental units, private philanthropies and doctors working without fees, workmen's compensation, etc. In a study performed for the Social Security Administration, Regina Lowenstein of Columbia University found that 17 percent of the hospital admissions of persons sixty-five and over in the year from the spring of 1965 to the spring of 1966, i.e., just before Medicare went into effect, were provided without bills being presented to the patient. Of the hospital bills paid for or by the elderly in that period, private insurance paid for 61.6 percent, while 38.4 percent were paid directly by the recipients.[5]

These observations bring us to an important characteristic of Medicare: It provides uniform benefits to all who are enrolled regardless of need. A millionaire has the same right to "free" hospitalization as a pauper, up to the limits indicated earlier, and the same is true for all those in between. From the patient's point of view, once the initial deductible is paid, there is little reason to economize on at least the first sixty days of hospitalization. Similarly SMI after the first deductible is met, sharply reduces the cost of seeing a doctor.

That Medicare would be popular with its recipients was anticipated by all. What Congress did not expect was the rapidity with which costs of Medicare zoomed upward beyond all earlier expectations. It is instructive, for example, to contrast the estimates made in 1965 of Hospital Insurance benefit payments in the years ahead with the actual amounts paid out. The discrepancies are so large that it makes little difference that the years in the table below are calendar years in the case of the initial estimates and fiscal years for the actual figures.[6] (See page 130.)

Why were such egregiously bad forecasts made? The main reason was simply that nobody involved had anticipated the sharp rate of medical care cost increases, especially hospital cost increases, that would be set off by Medicare and Medicaid. Yet once the program had been instituted, it could not be repealed, however much it cost. The imperatives of practical politics assured that. Hence the Congressmen, most unhappily, had to vote ever larger appropriations to

Year	Advance Estimate of Benefit Payments* (billion dollars)	Actual Benefit Payments**
1967	2.2	2.5
1968	2.4	3.7
1969	2.6	4.7
1970	2.9	4.8
1971	3.1	5.4
1972	3.3	6.3***
1973	3.5	7.4***
1975	4.0	n.a.
1980	6.1	n.a.
1990	9.0	n.a.

* Calendar year basis.
** Fiscal year basis.
*** 1973 budget estimate.

help pay for these rocketing costs. Nevertheless a lesson was deeply burned into the Congressional consciousness: No major health benefits can be extended to the population without very careful consideration of the costs involved, including those costs likely to be generated by additional inflationary pressure on the medical system.

It was not only hospital and physician costs that went up with the advent of Medicare. So did use of facilities in short term acute hospitals, the most expensive institutional source of medical care. Dr. Lowenstein's study referred to above compared use of these facilities during a year before Medicare began with utilization during a year shortly after Medicare began. She found a 25 percent increase in the number of hospital days per enrolled person sixty-five and over. The increases were particularly sharp for several categories. Persons over seventy-five, for example, increased their number of hospital days about 70 percent; Negroes increased their number of hospital days almost 50 percent; and old people living alone and having under $1,000 annual income more than doubled their number of hospital days.

These increases in utilization were short term effects, taking place in the transition period immediately before and after Medicare. One might explain them, as some have, in terms of a backlog of needed care in the elderly population which many persons could not afford before Medicare. There is undoubtedly some basis for this belief. Dr. Lowenstein's study found that the rate of cataract surgery more than doubled in the transition period she studied and the rate at which gall bladder operations were performed tripled. But the trend toward higher utilization of hospitals has continued since the transitional period. Between fiscal year 1967 and 1971 the number of hospital admissions per thousand persons enrolled under Medicare increased from 266 to 309, or better than 15 percent. Between 1967 and 1969 there was a 10 percent increase in the average length of hospital stay. The result was that just between 1967 and 1969 the total number of hospital days paid for by Medicare jumped almost 25 percent. But then alarmed Medicare officials slammed on the brakes, demanding tighter control of hospital utilization. The result was that the average length of stay in the hospital declined about 7 percent between fiscal year 1969 and fiscal year 1971. This drop more than compensated for the increased rate of Medicare hospital admissions. In fiscal 1971, as a result, Medicare paid for about 78 million days of hospital care as compared with 61.7 million days in 1967 and 81 million in 1969.[7]

Was all this vast amount of hospitalization necessary?

Most of it undoubtedly was necessary and justified. But there have been significant abuses, too. Frequently old people who have recovered from an illness or a bout of surgery properly treated in a hospital don't have anywhere to go or anyone to take care of them afterward. With the tightening of Medicare regulations on the use of extended care facilities, the tendency in some areas, for humanitarian reasons that are thoroughly understandable, is to keep them in hospitals, thus providing expensive custodial care. The problem involved is social, not medical, but the availability of seemingly free or cheap hospital care encourages the people involved to use the Medicare mechanism to meet the need.

Another source of concern arises from the sharp increase in the number of admissions per thousand persons sixty-five or over. The Lowenstein study estimated that in the year just preceding the beginning of Medicare there were 230 hospital admissions per thousand people sixty-five and over; by fiscal 1971 Medicare was experiencing 309 admissions per thousand enrollees. President Nixon's budget message in January 1972 estimated that by 1973 there would be 325 admissions per thousand enrollees. This suggests a 40 percent increase in the rate of hospital admissions in less than a decade. It is hard to believe that older Americans need hospitalization 40 percent more frequently in the early 1970s than they did in the mid 1960s. It is difficult not to suspect that some people covered by Medicare are simply demanding more hospital care because they see it as free or cheap.

Still more questions must be generated by the astonishingly wide variations of experience among different states. Here, for example, are the data on the number of hospital admissions per thousand Medicare enrollees in fourteen states, the seven lowest and the seven highest, in 1970: [8]

Lowest		*Highest*	
Maryland	222.5	North Dakota	476.3
New Jersey	229.8	Montana	439.7
Puerto Rico	239.8	South Dakota	409.4
New York	240.5	Colorado	400.0
Delaware	243.8	Texas	391.1
Rhode Island	245.7	Wyoming	386.4
Connecticut	246.9	Oklahoma	381.1

It seems highly improbable that the major differences in hospital admission rates shown above are related to actual differences in needs. Elderly persons in North Dakota and Montana can hardly get sick twice as often as persons the same age in Maryland and New Jersey. But there is a clue to help us explain this mystery. The clue is the fact that in general the states with the highest Medicare hospital admission rates are among the states having the highest ratio of community hospital beds to population. Conversely most of the states shown as having the lowest Medicare hospital admission rates belong to the group of states having the lowest ratio of community hospital beds to population.[9] The suspicion must arise that the great differences in Medicare hospital admission rates between these two groups of states mainly reflect differences in availability of hospital beds. Where beds are relatively abundant, they will be used more frequently than where they are less abundant. It is all another useful reminder of how elastic the concept of need can be with respect to a type of medical care whose recipients see it as "free."

The discussion above has been in terms of overall totals and global averages for the entire Medicare population. Additional insight is provided in the breakdown of use of Medicare funds by the amount of use. This has become possible only recently with the issuance of data for 1967, the first full calendar year of Medicare operation. It turns out that in 1967 only about one-third—34.5 percent to be exact—of the Medicare population benefited from that program's funds. Less than 7 percent of the Medicare population was reimbursed for $1,000 or more of medical expenses. But this relatively small group of approximately 500,000 people accounted for two-thirds of all Medicare reimbursements in 1967.[10] Many of the more than 6.5 million Medicare enrollees who received less than $1,000 in reimbursements during 1967 could presumably have afforded to pay their medical costs from their own or their children's resources.

Medicare's accomplishments in making first class medical care more available to the elderly sick are genuine and important. But it makes no differentiation among its beneficiaries between those who can afford to bear all or a substantial portion of their health costs and those who cannot. It treats identically people who are in very different situations, offering the same benefits to the aged person who has no resources beyond the monthly social security check and to the equally aged person whose resources include substantial savings, a good private pension, and affluent children.

Society's resources are limited. Money that is used for nonessential purposes—such as paying small medical bills for persons who can afford to pay those bills themselves—in Medicare is money that cannot be used for more essential needs elsewhere. One example is the care of the elderly in state mental institutions, a type of long term care that Medicare does not cover. Here is how Dr. Naomi R. Bluestone of New York City recently described the conditions prevailing in the geriatric wards of a mental hospital that is by no means the worst in the country:

Filth. Mice. Roaches. Garbage on the stairs and trash in the nurses' stations. No sheets, no underwear, no blankets in the winter. No furniture for patients save beds, and broken odds and ends. No page system. No telephone directory. No policy manuals. Rotted plumbing. Unpalatable food. One functioning elevator for one thousand patients on seventeen floors. One wheelchair ramp for the entire hospital. No electroencephalograph for the entire hospital. One dietitian for three thousand patients . . . Inadequate staff. Shattered morale. Employe theft. Patient theft. Elderly feeble beaten by young psychotics. Inability to protect patients from employe reprisals. Unexplained fractures during the night. Nonexistent charts. Physicians who speak a foreign tongue. Vital medications not given. Fatal bedsores, dehydration, coma, death.[11]

The senile elderly in mental hospitals are not the only people in American society whose medical needs are neglected. At the other end of the age spectrum mentally retarded and emotionally ill children are also frequently victims of inadequate care resulting from lack of funds. The tragic conditions at Willowbrook State Hospital in New York excited nationwide consternation when they were publicized in early 1972 but they are not unique either. With these and other genuine crisis areas in American medicine so desperately in need of resources, why should elderly Americans who can afford to pay small and moderate medical bills have those bills paid for by the government? The cynical will say that most old people who stand to benefit from Medicare can and do vote, while the senile elderly and retarded children cannot vote.

MEDICAID

No charge is made more frequently and more emotionally against the American medical system than the accusation that it neglects the poor. The fact that there are few private physicians in ghetto areas is usually interpreted by the critics as meaning that the poor have no, or almost no, access to the medical care they need. Those reaching this conclusion seemingly forget that, long before the modern welfare state, American medicine—physicians and hospitals alike—had a great and real tradition of providing charity care. A widespread popular belief once held that the only people who could afford first class care were the very rich and the very poor. And since the beginning of the American welfare state in the 1930s ever-increasing emphasis has been placed by the United States Government and by many state and local governments upon providing medical aid for the poor. Moreover the great migration of blacks from the South to the North has moved millions of the black poor from areas where medical resources are relatively scarce to areas where medical resources are relatively abundant.

The available statistics make evident that the usual stereotypes in this area are badly misleading. Over the past decade low-income Americans have regularly received more hospital care on the average than high-income Americans, and the margin of that superiority has been increasing rather than decreasing. By 1969 low-income Americans were receiving more physician visits per capita than either middle-income or high-income Americans. It is hard to avoid the conclusion, therefore, that poor people in this country have and have had much more access to the medical system than is usually supposed. Let us look at the data, first on persons hospitalized per thousand population and then on physician visits per capita.[12] (See page 137.)

These data do not prove, nor are they cited here to prove, that all the poor get adequate medical care. (Presumably the poor are sicker than other Americans on the aver-

	1962*	1966*	1968
	(persons hospitalized per 1,000 population)		
Low-income	94.7	106.6	114.5
Middle-income	97.6	100.9	95.4
High-income	86.7	88.9	81.8
Ratio, low-income to high-income	1.09	1.20	1.40

    * Fiscal year

	1964*	1967*	1969
	(physician visits per capita)		
Low-income	4.3	4.3	4.6
Middle-income	4.5	4.2	4.0
High-income	5.1	4.6	4.3
Ratio, low-income to high-income	0.84	0.93	1.07

    * Fiscal year

age, and therefore need even more medical attention than they get—or at least so it can be argued.) Nevertheless, awareness of the facts in the tables presented above may promote a re-examination of the most simplistic stereotypes.

The latest major chapter in the long history of this country's many efforts to improve the health care of the poor has been written by Medicaid or, to use its formal name, Title XIX of the Social Security Amendments of 1965. While Medicare has generally been approved in public discussion, Medicaid has had a generally bad reputation, and words like "muddle" and "chaos" are often used to characterize it. There seems wide agreement that Congress, when it enacted Medicaid, had little understanding of the consequences that would follow, particularly the great cost of the program and the opportunities it would provide for corruption and abuse.

One root of the Medicaid program derived from the earlier programs of federal grants to the states to help finance medical care for the poor. A second root came from the desire of Congressional and other reformers to create a "one class" system of medical care for poor and rich alike in this country, to permit the poor to enter the "mainstream" of American medical care with the federal, state, and local governments paying the bill. Unfortunately, Congress failed to foresee the fiscal consequences, especially at the state and local level, of the open-ended and potentially extremely generous program enacted at that time. Certainly there was no idea in Congress in the mid–1960s that Medicaid, if fully implemented, could cover the medical expenditures of 35 million people at a cost of $20 billion annually, as Professors Rosemary and Robert Stevens of Yale University estimate.[13]

Technically, Medicaid is a program which provides federal matching grants to states to induce them to set up medical assistance programs for welfare recipients and also for the "medically indigent," defined as persons with incomes above the welfare level but less than some higher amount. The legislation set some minimum requirements for types of services to be provided but it permitted each state to decide what medical services it wanted to finance. The legislation set no upper limit on the top income to be used to define the "medically indigent." In effect the states were given blank checks on the federal treasury to help finance medical care for the poor by paying for their hospital, doctor, and other medical care bills. The idea was to get rid of

charity medicine and enable the poor to get treatment as
private patients on a par with the middle and upper classes.
The goal was a heady one, defined in Section 1903 (e) of
Title XIX as assuring the "furnishing by July 1, 1975, [of]
comprehensive care and services to substantially all individuals who meet the plan's eligibility standards with respect to income and resources, including services to enable
such individuals to attain or retain independence or self-
care."

The goal was certainly generous, humanitarian, and
noble. In practice, too, it should be emphasized, Medicaid
has undoubtedly helped large numbers of poor and near-
poor people to receive more and better medical care than
they would have gotten without this program. We have suggested earlier that Medicaid may have been a significant
factor in helping bring about the sharp reduction in infant
mortality rates this country has enjoyed since the
mid–1960s.

Why then has Medicaid aroused so much controversy and
bitter opposition?

First, coming into effect simultaneously with Medicare,
Medicaid was part of the federally financed and federally
sponsored upsurge in effective demand for medical care
that fueled the great health care cost inflation of
1965–1971. It is worth emphasizing again that in enacting
both these programs Congress did nothing to increase simultaneously the nation's resources for meeting the new
effective demand that Congress placed on the market.

Second, some states, notably, but not exclusively, New
York and California, provided much more generous benefits than Congress had originally envisaged. In New York
the unexpected development was a high income ceiling for

the medically indigent. Thus originally a New York family
of four persons with an annual income of $6,000 was eligi-
ble for Medicaid benefits, while a household of ten persons
was eligible for Medicaid if it had an income of $11,000 or
less.[14] This generous eligibility standard roused a storm of
hostility in upstate New York where incomes are much
lower than in New York City; some local authorities
claimed up to 70 percent of their population would be eligible for Medicaid. Moreover, some county officials feared
their counties would be bankrupt since counties are required to pay a quarter of the Medicaid cost. Overall, it became apparent that 8 million New Yorkers, almost half the
state's population, would be eligible for Medicaid benefits.
Governor Nelson Rockefeller initially hailed the New
York Medicaid legislation as "the most significant social
legislation in three decades" but he was soon on the defensive and before many years were past he was helping lead
the fight to cut Medicaid as part of a frantic effort to save
his state from bankruptcy.[15]

In California, where only 13 percent of the population
was made eligible for Medicaid, problems were created by
the broad range of medical benefits included in the program and the elimination of earlier requirements that the
poor could only be cared for in county hospitals and clinics. This meant that the conventional medical system received a great influx of new paying customers, and Medicaid costs went up steeply and quickly.

New York and California were the extremes and the situation differed markedly in other states. The precipitous rise
of Medicaid costs is shown by the data below, and these
costs had to be met from taxation at the federal, state, and
local government levels: [16]

Fiscal Year	Vendor Medical Payments (billion dollars)
1965	1.4
1966	1.7
1967	2.5
1968	3.7
1969	4.6
1970	5.2
1971	6.5

These rapidly expanding costs, about half of which were paid by the federal government, quickly set off efforts to close the spigot at least partially. Thus 1967 amendments passed by Congress set top income limits for the medically indigent, forcing a number of states, including New York, to reduce the number of persons eligible for Medicaid. Many states thereafter also began cutting the medical services they would pay for, insisting upon tighter utilization review or pre-clearance for certain types of service. In the early 1970s, as unemployment rose under the impact of the depression, the number of persons eligible for Medicaid and using it rose sharply despite all efforts at limitation. The result, in state after state, was intense political battling between those who sought to economize on Medicaid and those who sought to keep its benefits intact and available to the largest possible number of recipients.

Third, some of the poor were brought into the mainstream of American medicine by Medicaid. They became private patients of able doctors and dentists and were operated on in some of the country's best hospitals. But many others among the poor did not get such benefits. They went to the doctors available in the slums—and since there were and are few of them, these doctors were flooded with patients—or to the clinics they had been accustomed to patronizing. Medicaid did encourage some doctors to move to the slums and ghettoes because practice there could be immensely profitable, especially for an unscrupulous minority who had no qualms about treating a huge volume of patients superficially and thereby earning a great deal of money.

As reports began to be published about physicians receiving large incomes—in some cases over $100,000 annually—from Medicaid practices in the ghettoes, the public impression grew that the program was a medical and dental gold mine. The result was public and official disillusionment which produced tighter bureaucratic controls and more paperwork, as well as efforts to cut fees to providers. These changes in turn tended to make Medicaid work less and less attractive to many health professionals and in many areas only a minority of doctors and dentists were willing to take on Medicaid patients. The effective New York City fee of four dollars for an office visit, for example, was hardly attractive for anyone wishing to give quality medical or dental care, both of which require time.

The attitude of many physicians serving Medicaid patients was stated in 1969 by the president of the black physicians' organization, the National Medical Association, Dr. Julius W. Hill. He complained, "I get so disgusted when I submit a bill and am treated like a suspect or criminal." Dr. Hill defended the doctors in the slums, saying this physician "is not getting the recognition he deserves. He is not getting the pay he deserves, so that what he is doing is almost a labor of love, and he is treating on the average about 60 patients a day. This is too many. You can't attract doctors to the ghetto when they don't get the pay they should." [17]

In Washington, D.C., there was a furor in April 1972 when it was revealed that fifty-four physicians, each of whom had gotten over $20,000 in payments from Medicaid in 1971, had together collected nearly half the total amount Medicaid paid physicians in Washington that year. The D.C. Medical Society announced that it would investigate four doctors who had received an average of nearly $100,000 each from Medicaid in 1971. One of the four under investigation, a black physician, noted that most of the doctors involved were black and accused the city government, the medical society, and the news media of racism. "Someone is actually appalled that a black doctor should make more than $100,000 a year," the doctor charged. Another physician being investigated in this matter asserted he was one of the very few psychiatrists, perhaps the only one in some heavily black Washington areas, willing to treat Medicaid patients. "These are the poor. I should be praised," he argued when asked about the $106,835 he had received in 1971 from Medicaid.[18]

Publicity about the large amounts received by physicians and others from Medicaid or Medicare often carries an implication of wrongdoing for which there may be no justification. One point involved was made well by William Raspberry, the black columnist of the *Washington Post,* in commenting on the criticism of high earnings by black physicians who treated Washington Medicaid patients. Mr. Raspberry wrote, "But if they [the black doctors involved] are making good money because they are providing good service to people who never had it before, what is wrong with that?" His question is an excellent one, worth consideration in contexts far beyond the one he considered in writing his comment. Moreover the public focus on money received from the government is a focus on gross income. A physician doing a good job in a ghetto would have to have assistance, employing aides hired to help him treat a large number of patients by taking electrocardiograms and X-rays, performing laboratory tests, etc. Where this is done, net income would be substantially less than gross income. Finally, a case can be made for government subsidy, if necessary, to encourage physicians to locate in ghetto areas and to practice good medicine despite the physical dangers and other special problems there.

These considerations suggest that evaluation of some of the publicity regarding Medicaid abuses is more complex than may appear at first sight. Nevertheless, there is no question but that some profiteering, and even some fraud, has taken place. But the abuses frequently come from the patients, too. Describing the problem, one Washington, D.C., physician has explained that he stopped seeing Medicaid patients in the black area where he works because they were "unfair to doctors." He asserted that many of the Medicaid patients who used to flock into his Southeast Washington office had "ailments they could have taken aspirin for. They demanded X-rays, prescriptions, and being sent to the hospital unnecessarily. They asked for medicine for friends or relatives and sometimes they even lent their Medicaid identification card to other people who weren't in the program so they could get free care." Another Washington doctor told the local medical society, "I joined Medicaid because I thought it was the right thing to do. Patients I used to treat free now want more frequent visits which they don't need and [they] bug me on the phone." And some doctors, the society discovered, found it simpler to treat Medicaid patients free of charge, feeling that the small fee they might get from Medicaid was not

worth the work, trouble, and aggravation associated with
submitting a Medicaid payment claim.[19]

Another view of Medicaid's troubles was given in late
1971 by Dr. Stephen N. Rosenberg, the deputy executive
medical director of New York City's Medicaid program:

> Medicaid was founded on the supposition that if doctors could
> make a living in areas where poor people live, they would move in.
> A good many did just that.
>
> Then the legislature cut back fees 20 percent, cut down on the
> number of eligibles and required patients to pay 20 percent of their
> doctor's bill. That pushed the practitioner to the edge, and perhaps
> over it. Doctors seldom collect that 20 percent. The fee now for a
> repeat visit to a general practitioner is $4 and change. Doctors feel
> it's demeaning to ask a patient for 80 cents, which he usually can't
> pay anyway. Should a doctor wear a change-maker, like a Good
> Humor man?
>
> So we find doctors who try to make up income by seeing 70 pa-
> tients a day, which means they give maybe six minutes to each.
> How much has the system pushed the doctor into that?

Dr. Rosenberg noted the perverse effects of Medicaid efforts to economize by cutting physician fees: "If a specialist
can treat a patient in his office, and we have cut his fee
from $16 to $8, he sends the patient over to the hospital
where we have to pay $40 per outpatient visit." [20]

The conventional liberal wisdom today is that Medicaid's
problems prove how obsolete private medical practice in
the United States is. Some liberals have welcomed the muddle and chaos of Medicaid as prods forcing the United
States toward a more "rational" medical system. Usually
that more "rational" medical system is depicted as prepaid
group practice, to which we shall turn in the next chapter.

But this is simplistic, naive thinking. What the Medicaid
semifiasco has shown above all is how poorly Congress and
state officials coped with the problem of providing medical

service for the poor. That failure is hardly encouragement to have these same legislators and bureaucrats expand further their maladroit intervention into the American medical system. The basic flaw of Medicaid as originally conceived was that it gave no incentives for economy to either the buyer or the seller of medical services. The more services a seller provided—for example, the more patients a ghetto doctor or dentist saw—the more money he made. But the patients, the Medicaid beneficiaries, had no reason to economize either since it cost them nothing to go to a doctor, enter a hospital, or have the dentist work on their teeth. On the contrary, more than a few Medicaid patients learned how to use that mechanism to satisfy nonmedical needs, for example by getting a podiatrist to "prescribe" ordinary shoes or taking an unnecessary prescription to a druggist and exchanging the prescription for cash amounting to, say, half the sum the pharmacist would be compensated for the medication. This was the worst of all possible worlds in terms of any rational use of resources. The original Medicaid system invited numerous abuses because it had built-in incentives for needless, wasteful utilization. It was a hypochondriac's heaven and an unscrupulous health service provider's paradise. Only after much money had been spent were drastic measures taken to improve the situation, measures that brought new problems.

There was another gross failure of imagination in Medicaid as originally conceived. If the poor of America were to get quality medical and dental care, the resources to deliver such care had to be provided. In the medical wastelands that are the ghettoes, with few physicians and dentists, more than money was and is needed for quality care. The few dozen OEO neighborhood health centers were and are inadequate to meet the needs. A rational effort to help the poor would begin by directly promoting the movement of needed personnel and facilities into the areas that are predominantly inhabited by welfare recipients.

Finally, Medicaid has forced the country to face the question of how much medical care is a human right. Is a person entitled to visit a doctor every time he has a headache or a stomach ache, or does his human right to medical care begin only when he has a genuinely serious illness? The limitations on access to hospital care, physicians, etc., that have been introduced to try to cope with the Medicaid expenditure explosion are an initial effort to come to grips with this important question. Those who bring nothing to this area but the slogan "Health care is a human right," are of no help. Society is not rich enough to give free of any direct charge all of the medical care everybody might want. That which is "free" and scarce—like medical care resources—must be rationed in some noneconomic fashion, and there is no simple, abuse-proof method on which to base rationing in this complex and sensitive area.

Medicaid does not prove that the American medical system must be radically reorganized. All it proves is that ill-conceived legislation can bring fiscal woes. In any case the health problems of the poor are not curable primarily through the medical system. Much of the money wasted on Medicaid could have been used more wisely to provide adequate nutrition and decent housing for those who need them. Those who look to Congress for new legislation to reform the American medical system radically should temper their enthusiasm by contemplating the costs and waste brought about by Medicare and Medicaid. As Professor William B. Schwartz of Tufts University has written, "the Medicare-Medicaid legislation has simply led to a redistribution of medical services—the poor and aged seeing the physician a little more frequently but everyone else seeing him less. The result has been, first, a staggering rise in costs as the newly insured have used their medical dollars to compete for a larger share of a fixed supply of services, and, second, ever longer queues as physician time has become a limiting factor in health care delivery." [21]

In the animated discussion of national health insurance during the early 1970s, the media and the political scene have for the most part been dominated by the worst proposals. The advocates of greatly extending the area of "free" medical care through a system of comprehensive national health insurance have disseminated horror stories about the American medical system, as well as Utopian fairy tales about the benefits their proposals would bring. There has been a dearth of sophisticated commentary and criticism to point out that adoption of overambitious measures such as the Kennedy bill could well worsen the medical care available to Americans by flooding the system with eager customers for "free" care.

An intelligent effort to restructure the present American medical payment system would have two objectives: First, to discourage abuse of the medical system by those who have no real need and by those who overuse hospital resources because their insurance makes hospital care seem "free." Second, to provide maximal help to victims of serious illness so as to protect families against financial disaster from catastrophic illness. Much of today's medical insurance operates perversely against these two objectives. It encourages resort to expensive medical care for relatively trivial complaints, while halting financial protection usually far short of the level to which bills can run in many cases of heart or kidney disease, cancer, stroke, psychiatric illness, etc. In effect those who need help most are denied it, while those who least need help are encouraged to take it bountifully.

Congress could do much to remedy this situation by enacting into law two provisions governing health insurance, a prohibition against front end medical insurance and introduction of some type of compulsory catastrophic illness insurance. The latter would be relatively cheap since, while every working class and middle class family lives in dread of bankruptcy from catastrophic illness, the actual incidence is, happily, very low. (There would have to be limits on the catastrophic insurance, of course, some mechanism, for example, for deciding at what point an eighty-year-old human being in a coma should have the respirators and other equipment keeping him physically alive turned off.) Many of the horror stories about American medicine disseminated by advocates of socialized or semisocialized medicine turn out to be cases where the only problem is the absence of catastrophic illness insurance rather than any iniquity of American hospitals, physicians, nurses, etc.

An ingenious proposal for a rational health insurance system has been advanced by Professor Martin S. Feldstein of Harvard University. Some features of his scheme are open to dispute, of course, but it seems worthwhile to present the core of his idea, which is a significant contribution to the current debate:

My proposal is extremely simple: major risk insurance (MRI) and government guaranteed postpayment loans. Every family would receive a comprehensive insurance policy with an annual direct expense limit (i.e., deductible) that increased with family income. A $500 "direct expense limit" means that the family is responsible for the first $500 of medical expenses per year but pays no more than

$500 no matter how large the year's total medical bills. Different relations between family income and the direct expense limit are possible. For example, the expense limit might start at $300 per year for a family with income below $3,000, be equal to 10 percent of family income between $3,000 and $8,000, and be $800 for incomes above that level. . . . The key feature is an expense limit that is large in comparison to average family spending on health care but low relative to family income. The availability in addition of government guaranteed loans for the postpayment of medical bills would allow families to spread expenditures below the expenses limit over a period of a year or even more.

Professor Feldstein points out that his MRI could be improved by introducing a coinsurance feature above a basic deductible—set lower than indicated above. As he notes, "This would make consumers cost sensitive over a wider range of expenditures without increasing the maximum risk to which they are exposed." His scheme deserves to be debated seriously, not least because its objectives of making consumers more cost conscious and giving them incentives for economy in medical care are essential if the continued large scale waste of resources is to end.[22]

NOTES

1. *Medical Care Costs and Prices: Background Book*. Social Security Administration, Office of Research and Statistics, January 1972, p. 96.
2. *American Medical News,* February 7, 1972.
3. Richard N. Rosett and Robert L. Berg, "Health Insurance: The High Cost of Violating Sound Principles" (manuscript).
4. Herbert E. Klarman, "Policy Alternatives for Controlling Health Service Expenditures," paper delivered at the annual meeting of the American Economic Association, December 28, 1970.
5. Regina Lowenstein, "Early Effects of Medicare on the Health Care of the Aged," *Social Security Bulletin,* April 1971.
6. SOURCES: The advance estimates are the intermediate cost estimates given in Robert J. Meyers, *Medicare.* Homewood Ill.: Richard D. Irwin, 1970, p. 200. Actual benefit payments are taken from various government sources, especially Special Analysis K accompanying President Nixon's January 1972 budget message to Congress.
7. Howard West, "Five Years of Medicare—A Statistical Review," *Social Security Bulletin,* December 1971.
8. U.S. Social Security Administration, Office of Research and Statistics, *Medicare Fiscal Years 1967–1970 Selected State Data.* Washington, D.C., 1971, *passim.*
9. *Basic Facts on the Health Industry.* Prepared for the use of the Committee on Ways and Means by the staff of the Committee on Ways and Means. Washington: U.S. Government Printing Office, 1971, p. 49.
10. West, *op. cit.,* pp. 25–27.
11. Naomi R. Bluestone, "Old Ones Go On the Discard Pile," *New York Times,* April 8, 1972, p. 29.
12. Charles L. Schultze, Edward R. Fried, Alice M. Rivlin and Nancy H. Teeters, *Setting National Priorities The 1973 Budget.* Washington, D.C.: The Brookings Institution, 1972, pp. 224–25.
13. Rosemary Stevens and Robert Stevens, "Medicaid: Anatomy of a Dilemma," *Law and Contemporary Problems.* Spring, 1970, p. 390.
14. Mark V. Pauly, *Medical Care at Public Expense.* New York: Praeger Publishers, 1971, p. 107.
15. Stevens and Stevens, *op. cit.,* pp. 366–367.

16. Alfred M. Skolnik and Sophie R. Dales, "Social Welfare Expenditures, 1970–1971," *Social Security Bulletin,* December 1971, p. 5.
17. *New York Times,* August 17, 1969.
18. *Washington Post,* April 8, 1972.
19. *Ibid.,* June 25, 1971.
20. Jay Nelson Tuck, "Medicaid: Why the Program Is Mortally Ill," *New York Times,* October 17, 1971.
21. William B. Schwartz, "Policy Analysis, Politics and the Problems of Health Care," *New England Journal of Medicine,* May 11, 1972, p. 1057.
22. Martin S. Feldstein, "A New Approach to National Health Insurance," *Public Interest,* Spring 1971.

CHAPTER VI

THE HMO ILLUSION

A new panacea for the nation's medical care problems is being aggressively recommended to Americans these days. Its very name—Health Maintenance Organization (HMO) —testifies to the Madison Avenue tactics being employed. If one believes the advocates for the HMO and its analogues in various bills before Congress, this is a real medical cornucopia. The HMO, we are told, will keep us healthy, extend our longevity, save our infants, guarantee we can get a doctor any time we need one, assure uniform first class care for everybody and do all this much more cheaply and efficiently than the "cottage industry" on which most of us now depend. We are advised to banish the old-fashioned private doctors—those "pushcart peddlers of modern medicine," according to the critics—and feast to our heart's delight in the new chrome and glass HMO medical supermarkets.

Both President Nixon and Senator Kennedy back the HMO concept, though they differ significantly about what HMOs should be and do. The Nixon Administration first introduced the term Health Maintenance Organization into current discussion and began pushing in Congress for government aid for establishment of HMOs throughout the country. The Administration also made plain the core of an HMO is a rather old idea, prepaid group practice on the model of the Kaiser-Permanente plans. Senator Kennedy has sought a much more ambitious version of the HMO and on March 13, 1972 he introduced his own bill to provide government backing for HMO creation and growth. Referring to hearings held by a subcommittee he heads, Senator Kennedy told the Senate that day, "We have heard from a great many very knowledgeable witnesses, who have almost unanimously endorsed the concept of HMOs." But even in the Kennedy eulogy there was a hint that matters might be a bit complicated. Even among these "very knowledgeable witnesses," he said, "substantial disagreement exists . . . as to the precise nature of an HMO." This is an important point to which we shall return.

The evening of the same day that Senator Kennedy introduced his HMO bill, there took place in the Washington Heights area of Manhattan a meeting called to consider forming a consumers council for the Washington Heights branch of the Health Insurance Plan of Greater New York (HIP). Second only to Kaiser-Permanente, HIP is one of the oldest and largest prepaid group practice organizations in the United States, a partial prototype of the HMO. It was the desire to learn HIP members' reaction to this partial HMO that induced me to attend the meeting.

Among the three hundred or so HIP members present that evening, there seemed to be no one with a kind word for the organization. Instead, person after person rose to voice complaints, often with marked bitterness and emotion. One frequently reiterated grievance was about the long waits to see the doctor. "You wait and wait and wait, and then you wait some more," one speaker complained. Several speakers declared that time and again HIP mem-

bers waiting for a doctor saw that same doctor's private patients being "smuggled in" ahead of his HIP patients. One
woman told of coming to the center after being in an automobile accident and waiting for four hours for an X-ray.
Finally, she told the audience, she despaired, left the HIP
center, went to a nearby private doctor and in "half an
hour" had been X-rayed, bandaged, and otherwise taken
care of. Another man spoke scathingly of the difficulty of
getting an annual physical examination from HIP, declar-
ing that he had found the process so time consuming and
degrading that "this year I went to a private doctor, paid
sixty dollars, got a physical exam and felt like a gentle-
man."

Other speakers had additional complaints: One told how
difficult it was to get a HIP doctor in an emergency, especially on Saturday afternoons and Sundays when the HIP
center was closed. One speaker complained about the laboratory which, he said, was open only four mornings a
week, so that people who needed much laboratory work
had to lose a great deal of time from their jobs. Others denounced the lack of privacy during examinations, with
clerks and other personnel wandering in and out of examinations, as well as the superficial way many HIP doctors
examined patients. The complaints left no doubt that a
vast gulf separated the grimy medical reality these HIP
members knew daily from the glowing visions of medical
paradise HMO propaganda paints.

Some weeks later I discussed the complaints I had heard
with a HIP official. He conceded the organization had
weaknesses and argued that it was trying to remedy them.
He questioned whether the persons who had attended the
meeting were representative and pointed out that thousands
of subscribers to the Washington Heights HIP group were
not present that evening, implying that they were a satisfied

"silent majority." I knew the last claim was exaggerated since I was personally acquainted with several dissatisfied HIP members in the area who had stayed away from the meeting because they were elderly and ailing. Obviously HIP has contented as well as unhappy members. But HIP has been in existence for a quarter of a century and has failed to convince more than a small fraction of New Yorkers of its superiority to fee for service medicine. And the complaints I had heard at the meeting proved that at least a significant minority of HIP members felt they were not getting good medical care in an atmosphere of dignity and convenience. I wondered why the HMO salesmen did not talk about the problems in HIP.

Was this HIP group unique in its complaints? It seems unlikely. In California in late 1971, for example, I spoke to officials of the California Council for Health Plan Alternatives, a group composed of unions that get health insurance benefits in their contracts. Speaking of Kaiser-Permanente, they damned it with faint praise. "It's the best we've got, but it's not very good." They complained of the long waits union members have to endure to see Kaiser-Permanente doctors and told horror stories of people with very serious illness who had allegedly not been properly treated. They voiced the suspicion that the amount of doctor time available for patients in Kaiser-Permanente might be declining because, they thought, the organization was giving more and more of its physicians opportunities to do research rather than see patients. They denounced rapidly rising Kaiser-Permanente rates in much the same terms others use complaining about rising physician fees.

Finally we may quote these jaundiced remarks about group medical practice by the late Dr. E. Richard Weinerman, who gained an intimate knowledge of the Kaiser-Per-

manente organization before he became Professor of Medicine and Public Health at Yale:

> The most successful groups are big and thus more efficient
> financially, more supportive of the physicians but more impersonal
> and fragmented to the patient. . . . The work rules, appointment
> systems, office hours, and telephone arrangements are all calculated
> to make life more bearable for the doctors, while the time and
> comfort of patients and nonmedical staff receive secondary consid-
> eration. . . . Physicians usually deal independently with patients;
> they are separated from colleagues in the routine of the day's work
> by rushed schedules, compartmentalized buildings, and the self-suf-
> ficient style of work of the solo practitioner. Group conferences,
> medical audits, and informal office consultations are, in my experi-
> ence, more common in the descriptive literature than in daily
> practice.[1]

But it would be just as unfair to focus only on the negative aspects of prepaid group practice and HMO as to con-
centrate only on the Utopian dreams of their most enthusiastic proponents. Prepaid group practice has existed long
enough in this country and has won enough support among
a section of both laymen and physicians to indicate that it
is one viable form of medical care delivery. One may be
skeptical of it as a panacea, as this writer is, and still agree
that it has a significant place in a pluralistic medical system
as one alternative for both patients and physicians. The situation would be quite different, of course, if this mode of
health delivery were to be imposed upon all Americans,
giving it a monopoly position that would collectivize all
physicians, all patients, and all health care delivery. So long
as prepaid group practice has competition and all involved
in it have alternatives, it can and will make a significant
contribution to American medical care. But this mode of
medical service is not necessarily superior to that offered by
private physicians, a fact evidenced by what Professor

Anne R. Somers has called the "less than dramatic rise in enrollment" of such schemes since their inauguration about thirty-five years ago. In 1968, Dr. Weinerman judged that prepaid group practice had experienced "neither clearcut success nor abject failure" in its long history, while in early 1971 Professor Somers estimated that depending upon how one defined prepaid group practice there were either 20–25 prepaid medical groups with less than 4 million members or 125 groups with about 8 million members. But even the latter accounted for only about 4 percent of the American population.[2]

It is true, of course, that legal barriers in some states have hindered the spread of prepaid group practice. Any believer in free competition must deplore these artificial limitations. But it seems significant that this type of medical organization has by no means proliferated everywhere in the many states where it is legal. There are serious difficulties to be overcome in creating and operating this type of medical organization, difficulties quite independent of legal problems.

Why then the present interest in expanded versions of prepaid group practice—under the name of Health Maintenance Organizations—and the widespread "gold rush" to get on the bandwagon, a "gold rush" in which medical schools, hospitals, and even some insurance companies are prominent? The answer arises originally from the Nixon Administration's concern about the rocketing cost of medical care under Medicare and Medicaid, as well as its search for an answer to Senator Kennedy's national health insurance program. The catalytic agent was apparently a Minnesota physician and medical services delivery planner Dr. Paul M. Ellwood, who convinced the Nixon Administration that the HMO concept was the answer. Dr. Ellwood has argued that this organizational form would bring new incentives to physicians to keep patients healthy, and to cure them as quickly and cheaply as possible when they get sick. In this way, HMO proponents believe these organizations would simultaneously improve the nation's health and cut medical care costs. In effect the argument is that in medical care it is possible to have one's cake and eat it too.[3]

Before examining Health Maintenance Organizations in detail, it will be useful to consider their predecessors at least briefly. The existing organizations for delivery of medical care which HMO advocates have suggested can be developed into health maintenance organizations are at least four in number: Prepaid group practices, medical foundations, hospital-based medical services usually growing out of expansion of hospital emergency and clinic services, and OEO neighborhood health centers. Let us look at each of these in turn.

The most important prepaid group practice organizations in this country are the Kaiser Foundation Health Plan (Kaiser-Permanente), Health Insurance Plan of Greater New York (HIP), the Group Health Cooperative of Seattle, the Community Health Association of Detroit, whose financial troubles recently required its reorganization, and the Group Health Association of Washington, D.C. The table below gives the membership of these organizations: [4]

Year	Total	Kaiser-Permanente	HIP	Seattle	Detroit	Wash. D.C.
		(thousands of members)				
1964	2,061	1,168	694	76	69	54
1970	3,127	2,167	672*	143	70	75

* In 1970 HIP also enrolled 92,000 welfare and Medicaid recipients, who are not included in this figure.

Prepaid group practices have grown unevenly. Between 1964 and 1970, Kaiser-Permanente almost doubled its membership as did the Group Health Cooperative in Seattle. Washington's Group Health Association membership grew about 40 percent. HIP actually lost members in its conventional plan and grew only by adding welfare and Medicaid recipients. Detroit's Community Health Association remained essentially static in membership.

Kaiser-Permanente is a remarkable achievement, a monument to the ingenuity of its founder, Dr. Sidney Garfield, and to the generous backing of the late industrialist, Henry Kaiser, and the companies he controlled. Operating in California, Oregon, Hawaii, Cleveland, and Denver through eighteen legally separate organizational units, Kaiser-Permanente offers its members integrated medical care based upon availability of both physicians and hospitals. Three organizations are at the core of these arrangements: The Kaiser Foundation Health Plan, Inc., a nonprofit corporation that sells the basic medical service to groups of consumers and contracts with the two other organizations to deliver the promised services. The Permanente Medical Groups are mainly partnerships of physicians who provide all medically appropriate services in physicians' offices, in the hospital, and, to a small extent, in patients' homes. The Kaiser Foundation Hospitals is a nonprofit corporation that contracts with the Kaiser Foundation Health Plan to provide medical center facilities, i.e., inpatient hospital facilities, outpatient office facilities, and all other land, buildings, and equipment needed for a modern medical center. The Kaiser-Permanente formula includes prepayment, group practice, full time commitment by member physicians who may not moonlight elsewhere or pocket fees from private patients, and the availability of integrated facilities for both ambulatory and hospital care. The success of Kaiser-Permanente in the medical care marketplace provides an impressive example of the creative possibilities of private enterprise in a competitive situation. One may have serious reservations about Kaiser-Permanente, as this writer does, and yet recognize that it has made a valuable contribution toward a more pluralistic national medical system.

For contrast we may note that HIP is quite different. HIP itself is mainly only a brokerage organization that sells prepaid comprehensive medical, surgical, and diagnostic service packages to groups, especially to employees of New York City. Until recently it owned no hospitals, but it now owns one hospital, the 200–bed LaGuardia Hospital in Queens. Groups of physicians contract with HIP to provide medical services; the groups own their own centers and pay the costs of operating and staffing them. The physicians belonging to HIP groups—1,100 in early 1972—include only 30 percent who are full time. The remaining 70 percent are part time with HIP and have their own independent private practices as well. HIP members must have Blue Cross or other separate hospital insurance to cover their hospital stays, though HIP physicians will operate on members and otherwise provide medical service in hospitals at which HIP physicians have admitting privileges. Thus HIP has a more limited sphere of activity than Kaiser-Permanente and suffers some problems the Kaiser-Permanente organization does not have. We shall discuss later the complications that have arisen lately as HIP has sought to move toward the Kaiser-Permanente pattern.

We turn now to the medical foundations which were most active originally in California but which now seem to be spreading throughout the nation. In California, the creation of many of these foundations was the answer of doctors engaged in conventional medical practice to the appearance of Kaiser-Permanente competition in their area or to the threat of such competition. Medical foundations take many forms but the type of most interest to us might be called prepaid nongroup practices. In these a medical foundation will sell a contract to provide prepaid medical care to the employees or members of some organization—a corporation, a union, a governmental unit, etc. The individuals who become foundation subscribers are then entitled to get medical, surgical, diagnostic, and related services from the physicians who are affiliated with the foundation. As in HIP, foundation members' hospital costs must be insured separately through Blue Cross or some other insurer. The patient can choose his doctor from any of the foundation physicians and can change doctors when he pleases. The services provided the patient are paid for on a fee for service basis but the bill goes to the foundation rather than to the patient. The foundation has at least two controls over costs. Foundation physicians often agree to a maximum fee schedule and the foundation itself reviews the services provided to subscribers, retaining the right to refuse to pay for services it feels are unjustified. In an extremity when the bills for services to foundation subscribers exceed the income received from prepayment revenues, the physicians belonging to a foundation may have to accept a reduction in their payments proportional to the amount by which the foundation's income falls below the total of bills received. A further development, pioneered by the Sacramento Medical Foundation, is the so-called Certified Hospital Admissions Program (CHAP) under which the foundation reviews all except emergency hospital admissions in advance and rules out hospital admissions it regards as unnecessary. A foundation using the CHAP device has many of the controls over cost enjoyed by a prepaid group practice; the physician has greater freedom and independence of practice than in a prepaid group and the patient has a wider choice of physician than he would have in a closed panel prepaid group practice. On the other hand, some critics have argued that medical foundations are illegal collusive arrangements which set fees and limit competition among members. That accusation has never been sustained in court, however, and it seems obvious that competition between individual physicians persists among foundation members in a way it does not exist among physicians working full time for prepaid groups.

Finally the growth of patient visits to hospital emergency rooms and clinics—often by people who have no emergency but either have no regular doctor or are unable to reach their regular doctor—has led to increasing interest in the creation of hospital-based medical practices. Some eminent medical economists such as Nora Piore of Columbia University have urged that such arrangements be made the basis for a national medical care system. In any case there is rising interest among hospitals in becoming integrated deliverers of medical care, and the number of physicians accepting full time positions with hospitals for this purpose is growing. A hospital employing a staff of physicians could become a prepaid group practice center, or, to use the currently fashionable term, a Health Maintenance Organization.

In her recent study of this matter, Mrs. Piore argues ". . . hospital-based group practices offer what may be the only workable way to provide systematic medical service for large numbers of people who do not have and cannot establish a connection with private practitioners. It seems to be a feasible way to work out and substitute orderly medical arrangements for the present random and probably wasteful use of these hospital resources." Mrs. Piore notes that such use of hospitals may complement the OEO Neighborhood Health Center movement which has sought to provide comprehensive health care for the poor but which has grown much less than anticipated. As Mrs. Piore describes the situation, "The most dramatic effort to provide an alternative to the hospital clinic has been the Neighborhood Health Center movement. A major goal of the War on Poverty was to establish eight hundred such centers to provide care for 20 million urban poor estimated to be without adequate or satisfactory health services. Today, six years later, the forty OEO centers in operation offer service to about half a million registered persons and something like a million and a half visits a year." The OEO centers have had difficulties, both because of the special health problems of their clients and because of the effort to provide many services prepaid group practices do not provide, such as the employment of neighborhood health aides to go into poverty communities, find people who need medical care, and induce them to come to where they can obtain it. In addition, there have been some bitter political battles over community control of particular health centers. But of course Neighborhood Health Centers, if properly financed, could also become Health Maintenance Organizations.[5]

With this background material stated, let us look more closely at the concept of Health Maintenance Organizations. Here is the Nixon Administration's definition as given in the Department of Health, Education, and Welfare's *White Paper* of May 1971: "HMOs are organized *systems* of health care, providing comprehensive services for enrolled members, for a fixed, prepaid annual fee. No matter how each HMO may choose to organize itself (and there are various models), from the consumer's viewpoint they all provide a mix of outpatient and hospital services through a single organization and a single payment mechanism." (italics in original) A footnote to this definition gives Kaiser-Permanente as "an example of an HMO." But we have already noted earlier Senator Kennedy's observation that the matter is not so simple and that many experts who recommend HMOs disagree sharply about what these organizations are or should be.

Nevertheless, the logic of the HMO argument is easily stated. Under an HMO an individual's health becomes the concern of a medical organization, not merely a single doctor. The HMO gets a fixed advance payment for each patient. Therefore, it is argued, the HMO has a strong incentive to keep the patient healthy and to cure him quickly and cheaply when he does get sick. The HMO that does a good job, it is held, will make money. The HMO that somehow or other cannot prevent its patients from getting sick and cannot find quick easy ways to cure its sick patients will lose money.

Moreover, HMO proponents argue, this is not merely theory. They point to statistics from Kaiser-Permanente and some other prepaid group practice organizations to show that these systems are able to take care of their patients with fewer days of hospitalization per patient than Blue Cross-Blue Shield and other alternative non-HMO methods of financing medical care. The Nixon Administration 1971 *White Paper,* for example, cited studies showing that in HMO-type organizations there were only 744 hospital days per 1,000 enrollees each year as compared with 955 hospital days per 1,000 persons in non-HMO-type systems of medical care. It also cited Social Security Administration data showing "that some HMO's are saving as much as 15 percent on their elderly enrollees, in comparison with costs under traditional modes of practice." [6]

If these arguments were not enough, the Nixon Administration offered grants to organizations interested in starting HMOs. Under the leadership of President Nixon, it has made plain that it wants a rapid development of these organizations so that they will be available for 80 percent of the American people by the end of the 1970s. Needless to say, there has been no shortage of people willing to take government money to start organizing and researching HMOs in their localities. By April 1972 some 110 grants had been made for HMO planning and feasibility studies.

It will be argued here that the current Nixon-Kennedy enthusiasm for HMOs is misplaced or at the very least premature. Before beginning the examination of the Utopian promises, it is only fair to note that Kaiser-Permanente officials are much less starry-eyed than the propagandists who have had no experience with the actual problems of prepaid group practice. Addressing a conference of medical school representatives in early 1971, for example, the president of the Kaiser Foundation Health Plan and of the Kaiser Foundation Hospitals, Dr. Clifford H. Keene, referred pointedly to "our shortcomings" and said, "We ourselves don't see Kaiser-Permanente as a panacea. We do see it as *one valid solution* to some long standing problems. We do see it as an evolving method of organizing and delivering medical care which is intended to be responsive to the changing needs of the people it serves. We at Kaiser-Permanente are also impressed with the difficulties of altering existing patterns of medical care. We are aware of the talent, effort, and money needed to organize a medical care delivery system. . . ." [7] (italics in original)

Let us turn now to the roseate promises of the HMO advocates and see the grounds for skepticism that are provided by the cool light of reason and analysis. In doing so we should note the strong similarity in approach between the propaganda for HMOs and the manufacturer's instructions for taking care of one's automobile. Implicit in the whole HMO argument is the notion that the human body is something like an automobile. If we only service it properly at the required intervals, change the spark plugs, points and oil filters regularly, and otherwise take care of a car, it will normally give trouble-free operation for years.

Preventive maintenance may be the key to automobile health but it is inadequate for human beings who are much more complex than automobiles or other simple machines. The notion that HMOs can radically improve the health of people rests upon several misconceptions. For example, it exaggerates our knowledge of the causes of disease and the means of preventing them. It is true we can immunize people against diseases like smallpox and diphtheria. But those diseases have essentially been eliminated in this country or are only minor causes of illness and death. The main causes of death now are cancer, heart disease, and other degenerative ailments and our ignorance of these is still vast. There is no vast body of knowledge about how to prevent disease lying unused and available for application by a nationwide network of HMOs.

At this point the HMO advocates will no doubt want to counterattack. They will want to tell us about the great contribution HMOs can make to their patients' health by education, telling them to stop smoking, to keep their weight down, to exercise, to avoid alcoholism and drug addiction, and the like. Such health education is admirable, but similar advice is carried in the media every day. Is there any person who watches television, listens to the radio and reads newspapers and magazines who does not know that cigarettes, alcohol, and narcotics are harmful, that obesity cuts longevity and that exercise performed regularly is highly desirable? These facts are not secret. They have been and are shouted from the roof tops. The tragic fact is, however, that millions of Americans disregard this knowledge every day, even though they are aware that in the long run—or sometimes in the short run—they are injuring their health. The factors in American society and in the psyches of individual Americans that predispose our citizens to all their many health-destructive habits and practices are far too fundamental to be eliminated by routine health lectures or informational pamphlets received at an HMO. During World War II, I recall, every soldier and sailor in the United States armed forces was regularly and frequently lectured on the precautions to be followed to avoid contracting syphilis and gonorrhea. Nevertheless thousands of men in uniform disregarded the advice and became victims of venereal disease. Isn't the same result likely now? One must be optimistic indeed to believe that HMOs can dispel the despair which drives ghetto youngsters to heroin. Nor is it very much more likely that they can alter the lifestyles of many middle-aged Americans who overeat, smoke cigarettes, drink two Martinis or more daily, avoid exercise, and spend much of their free time sitting before a television set watching their favorite sports teams in action. It would require a genuine cultural revolution—not merely an abundance of HMOs—to induce Americans to give up juicy steaks, double ice cream cones, shrimp cocktails, and other delicious, but cholesterol-rich staples in the American diet.

But, the HMO advocates may counter, their concept removes the financial barrier to medical care. By encouraging people to come in for regular checkups and at the first sign of trouble, won't HMOs be able to catch diseases early, while they are still curable? Here, too, some fact is mixed with excessive optimism. The utility of regular physical examinations for adults under, say, forty-five is questioned by many medical authorities, though there is more likelihood that they will detect significant pathology at older ages. While the glare of publicity has focused on diseases detected early and cured, it must be remembered that there are many ailments about which medicine can do nothing even if they are detected relatively early. Such early discovery of incurable ailments may even be counterproductive because the psychic distress their discovery causes the sufferers is not compensated for by any increased likelihood of cure. Beyond that, the HMO—by combining health education and "free" access to physicians—may tend to encourage hypochondria and unnecessary physician visits and unnecessary laboratory and X-ray tests.

The problem of the hypochondriac in a "free" medical system is a central one. The matter is not theoretical, as can be seen in this comment from a Kaiser-Permanente official in the Oakland-San Francisco area:

> The role of the psychiatric department in Northern California has been interesting. We have attempted to develop a psychiatric service that would help the internist to screen or evaluate his patients—to tell him whether the patient is curable, whether he ought to keep on working with him from a somatic viewpoint or whether his complaints are going to keep one or two steps ahead of every suggested therapy. This approach to psychiatry, as an adjunct help to the internist, has been quite successful. We have had considerable help from them.[8]

The total or near-total elimination of any payment for the right to consult a physician tends to clog up any system of medical care. Here is the way the founder of the Kaiser-Permanente system, Dr. Sidney Garfield, put the matter in an article in the *Scientific American* in April 1970:

Elimination of the fee has always been a must in our thinking, since it is a barrier to early entry into sick care. Early entry is essential for early treatment and for preventing serious illness and complications. Only after years of costly experience did we discover that the elimination of the fee is practically as much of a barrier to early sick care as the fee itself. The reason is that when we removed the fee, we removed the regulator of flow into the system and put nothing in its place. The result is an uncontrolled flood of well, worried-well, early-sick and sick people into our point of entry—the doctor's appointment—on a first come, first served basis that has little relation to priority of need. The impact of this demand overloads the system, and, since the well and worried-well people are a considerable proportion of our entry mix, the usurping of available doctors' time by the healthy people actually interferes with the care of the sick.

Dr. Garfield's candid statement of the problem has made him a controversial figure among those who favor prepaid group practice. This pioneer, whose contribution in this area is now historic, has been accused of being opposed to prepaid group practice and in private conversation I have heard some people attack him cruelly. But a former California Health Commissioner, a well known advocate of reorganization of medical care, has tacitly conceded at least part of the Garfield argument by telling me, "The trouble with Kaiser-Permanente is they're too stingy. They just don't want to hire enough doctors." A young California physician who had spent a year working for Kaiser-Permanente in a "walk in clinic" told me in 1971, "Every time the gang of doctors who worked in our center got together for a bull session we talked about how wonderful it would be if we could charge $10 a visit so we could cut down the number of nuts and hypochondriacs."

Entirely independent support for Dr. Garfield's assertions has been provided recently by a former HIP physician, Dr. Bernard L. Albert, a Bronx, New York, internist. Writing in an April 1972 issue of *Medical Economics,* Dr. Albert declares, "it was my patients who drove me out of" HIP. Explaining that the bulk of his HIP patients were New York City employees who got membership free of charge as a fringe benefit, he declares "too many of them exploited it outrageously." A board certified internist, Dr. Albert became his HIP patients' family doctor. He describes the consequences in these terms:

I quickly discovered that to most of my patients, the term [family doctor] was roughly equivalent to "the family car." They felt that I belonged to them, and was at their beck and house call by day or night. As a result, the bulk of my practice was trivia medica. I did see a truly sick person now and then, but it was unusual for me to have a patient in the hospital. The really interesting cases I encountered—and almost my only medical challenges—were my private-practice referrals from outside doctors. Worse still, the trivia consumed so much time that I had to cut short patients who really needed me.

In a reply to Dr. Albert, Dr. George Brown, head of the HIP medical group to which Dr. Albert had belonged, wrote, "The fact that our patients are not reluctant to bring us their problems is what HIP prepaid practice and preventive medicine are all about. People go to a doctor because of a need, which is very real to the patient even if it's neurotic. If it is indeed a neurotic need—and we all draw our share of hypochondriacs—it's the doctor's job to relate to it, even if only as a good listener."

The Executive Director of the Northern California Permanente Medical Group has directly contradicted Dr. Garfield in public. The official, Dr. Cecil C. Cutting, has declared that "overutilization by members with psychosomatic problems has not been a serious problem." [9] But the writer of a study of the Kaiser-Permanente Health Plan, a study sponsored by the Henry J. Kaiser Foundation, gives a very different impression when he declares that Dr. Garfield offers no evidence for his charge "other than Permanente doctors' clinical impressions that 50 to 70 percent of their patients appear well." [10] The fact we noted earlier, that Kaiser-Permanente physicians prescribe so many analgesics and tranquilizers, also seems to speak in favor of Dr. Garfield's thesis.

It should be added that officials of a different prepaid medical care plan admit that they have some problem with hypochondriacs. Officials of the Sacramento Medical Foundation explained to me that when their records show a subscriber is going from doctor to doctor with the same hypochondriacal complaints they take effective action to assure that he will halt this abuse.

It can hardly be doubted that it is the economic arguments for the HMO form of medical care delivery that have seemed most persuasive to government officials. The HMO has been sold as a means of cutting costs. Washington has been impressed by figures alleging that hospital usage and total cost of care are lower in prepaid group practice than in conventional practice by fee for service doctors.

These economic arguments rest on shaky foundations, however. A number of eminent medical economists— perhaps most prominently Professor Herbert E. Klarman of New York University—have repeatedly questioned the adequacy and validity of the evidence for the alleged economic advantages of prepaid group practice. In a recent article in *Law and Contemporary Problems,* for example, Professors Judith R. Lave and Lester B. Lave of Carnegie-Mellon University commented: "Some years ago, group practice, especially prepaid group practice, was heralded as the solution to many cost (and quality) problems. Investigators liked what they saw in the Kaiser groups and attempted to persuade physicians to replicate this situation and to encourage the government to promote group practice. More recently, questions have been raised as to whether group practice itself really does result in a more efficient utilization of physicians and facilities. One may wonder whether the original investigators were guilty of trying to generalize from the experience of a prepaid group that had considerable constraints on its access to hospital beds." Let us look more closely at some of the reasons for the skepticism these specialists express about the alleged economic advantage of the prepaid group practice, and therefore, by implication, of the HMO.

First, almost all the prepaid group practice experience to date has been with carefully selected groups whose members enjoy better than average health. When Kaiser-Permanente contracts to provide care for West Coast longshoremen or New York City's HIP contracts to provide care for the city's policemen or firemen, they are taking on relatively elite populations from the health point of view. Such union groups consist of people in the prime of life and their children; they do not include the elderly, adults who are so sick that they cannot work or the very poor who are unemployed and suffer the pathologies of the ghetto. To extrapolate Kaiser-Permanente experience to the total population is an elementary statistical error. The unrepresentative character of the Kaiser-Permanente patient population has been explicitly recognized by that organization's medical economists. For example, Arthur Weissman and Richard Anderson have written: "Our membership is younger than the general population; 40 percent of our Northern California members are under twenty years of age while 4 percent are aged sixty-five and over. In contrast, 37 percent of the general population residing in the same area is under twenty years of age while 9 percent are sixty-five or over." [11] And it is the elderly who require the most medical care.

When I asked a Kaiser-Permanente planner in California what the motive was for Kaiser-Permanente's drive to expand, his answer was immediate: "As long as we keep expanding, our patient population won't get too old. If we remain static, our average patient's age will get older and older and then we'll be in trouble economically. This way every time we get a new union or a new factory, we get only the people who are working now and are in good health; not the retirees and the people who've had to quit because of a disabling disease." Such a consideration may be fine for an organization covering only a small percentage of Americans but there is no such easy out when providing HMO care for all Americans.

A second major point is overlooked by those who accept uncritically the HMO versus non-HMO comparisons given above. The available data on Kaiser-Permanente or HIP or other similar organizations' costs and hospitalization rates significantly understate the total cost of their patients' medical care. This is because many members of prepaid medical practice plans go outside their groups to get a portion— sometimes a very significant portion—of their medical care. Questioning an informal small sample of HIP and Kaiser-Permanente patients, I have found that there are at least two patterns of outside use of medical resources. Some people go to a fee for service doctor for relatively minor complaints, since they prefer to pay a fee and get prompt service rather than put up with the inconveniences of prepaid group practice; these people will turn to prepaid group practice for major surgery or serious illness that would involve heavy medical and hospital bills if obtained outside the prepaid group. There is also the exact opposite pattern. Some people use prepaid groups primarily for minor ailments where they don't care what doctor they get; when faced with life-threatening illness, they prefer to choose their own surgeon, internist, or other specialist and to be in the hospital of their choice, and for that freedom of choice they are willing to pay extra. No doubt there are other patterns. The fundamental point is that the statistics alleging the advantages of prepaid group practice need to be corrected to allow for this substantial understatement of the true total cost of their members' medical care. Such correction is rarely made.

The few clues that are available on the outside employment of medical care resources by prepaid group subscribers are suggestive and intriguing. Here, for example, is the revelation made in a book sponsored by the Henry J. Kaiser Foundation:

> A new KP consumer satisfaction study in Southern California . . . asked a random sample of Kaiser Plan members if "you or any member of your family had occasion to see any other doctor or use any other medical services" since becoming a Kaiser Plan member; 44 percent said "yes." This compared with a similar study in 1961 in which one-third of old members and one-half of new members said they had used outside services at some time.[12]

Professor John M. Glasgow of the University of Connecticut School of Medicine has recently surveyed the evidence on the supposed cost and other advantages of prepaid group practice and his reaction is hardly likely to comfort the enthusiasts. Insofar as this mode of organization may exhibit cost advantages, he notes, "it is not clear whether the cost experience . . . reflects the form of the organization, the composition of the patient population, the type of physician attracted to a group setting, the use of services outside the group, or some other factor. Consequently, arguments that the development of prepaid group practices will necessarily lead to improvements in the quality of care rendered, to innovative methods of delivery, or to huge savings in physician time and patient expense, which other practice forms by their very nature can not produce, would seem premature." He adds the further cautionary note that "it is not altogether clear how, should prepaid groups become a dominant organizational form, savings of the magnitude envisioned will be realized. Indeed, even without the inclusion of high risk groups, the rate of increase in medical expenditures of the Kaiser Health Plan, although less than that of Californians in total, is not much less than the rate of increase in the health sector as a whole. Kaiser Health Plan rates increased an average of from 6 to 8 percent a year from 1957 to 1966, and from 11 to 14 percent from 1966 to 1970. Moreover, an 18 percent increase was instituted in early 1971." [13] A Kaiser-Permanente vice president has published a similar cautionary warning against expecting cost miracles. The official, John J. Boardman, Jr., has written, "We do not operate in a world unto ourselves, free from external influences. We are not free from the inflationary spiral; we are as directly affected by certain external economic factors as anybody in the health care field. We compete in the same marketplace for personnel and buy our goods from the same vendors. We must consistently equal or exceed the standards of care in the community. Each new technological advance in medicine must be incorporated into the program as soon as it is generally available." [14]

For a better understanding of the economics of prepaid group practice, and therefore of an HMO, we need to look a little more deeply at the basic arrangements involved. In conventional fee for service arrangements, it can be argued, the doctor has an interest in maximizing the amount of work he does and is paid for, and the patient has an interest in minimizing the services he requires of a doctor and therefore pays for. In prepaid group practice, the tables are exactly reversed. Since the group is paid a fixed sum per patient, the medical group is interested in doing as little as possible and thus minimizing its costs per patient. The patient, on the other hand, has every incentive to maximize demands on the medical system since he pays no—or in some cases, very little—extra cost. It has been argued by HMO proponents that this means a prepaid group or an HMO has a great economic incentive to keep patients healthy. But looked at purely from a bookkeeping point of view, an HMO has an equally strong economic interest in having its seriously ill patients die quickly and inexpensively. Death is the ultimate economy. From the point of view of an HMO's finances, the patient who drops dead of a heart attack on the street is a blessing, while the cardiac patient who lingers on for months in intensive coronary care is a disaster since it may cost two to three hundred dollars a day to care for him adequately. This is not to argue that the personnel in prepaid groups are less compassionate and humane than physicians in fee for service practice. It is simply to note that expensive long term care is financially disadvantageous to a prepaid medical organization. If a complex and time consuming operation is likely to save a patient in, say, only 25 percent of all cases, the incentive for performing it is greater for a fee for service physician than for a physician in a prepaid practice.

Let no one doubt that prepaid group practices are very, very cost conscious. I was not surprised, for example, visiting a Kaiser-Permanente hospital in Los Angeles, to find a mimeographed announcement on a bulletin board warning nurses that their pay would be docked if they reported for work six minutes or more late. Kaiser-Permanente planners make no secret of their intense preoccupation with costs when they plan their facilities. They have every incentive to minimize the number of physicians, other personnel, and hospital beds available to their subscribers. The cost of such minimization is increased waiting time for patients wishing to consult a specialist or to enter a hospital for non-emergency surgery. But patients' waiting time does not cost a prepaid group anything—except in the area of consumer satisfaction—while the salaries and construction costs saved show up as pluses in its financial accounts.

Mr. Boardman, the Kaiser-Permanente vice president referred to earlier, has explained how this organization plans on the basis of statistical averages Historically, he notes, Kaiser-Permanente has regarded two hospital beds per 1,-000 members—a relatively low figure—as a desirable ratio. But in Southern California during 1961–1970 he reports, his organization was able to get by with slightly less than 1.8 beds per 1,000 members. In 1970 the overall average occupancy rate in beds for acute illnesses was 91 percent. During these years evidently, the Kaiser-Permanente hospitals were always full or nearly full so that the group's physicians were under extreme pressure not to hospitalize patients. Discussion of the cost of medical care tends to focus on the wasteful practice of hospitalizing patients unnecessarily; but in the situation described by Mr. Boardman one must wonder about the opposite error, whether some patients who should have been hospitalized were not. Certainly Mr. Boardman makes no bones about his belief that if more beds had been available his doctors would have hospitalized more people. As he puts the matter: "It is our firm conviction that if one has more beds than experience indicates is necessary to serve a given population, the utilization rate increases." [15] But it is the accountants who define what is "necessary."

This parsimony with hospital beds may be fine for Kaiser-Permanente finances and for the statistics HMO advocates like to quote, but patients may have a more jaundiced view of the matter. Here is how Greer Williams describes the situation in the book he did for the Henry J. Kaiser Foundation:

Bed utilization in the most active Kaiser hospitals impresses observers accustomed to a slower pace. Certain Kaiser Hospitals in the Los Angeles and San Diego areas in 1970 reported occupancy rates between 100 and 110 percent. Hospitals in the San Francisco Bay-Sacramento area have had similar crowding problems in the past.

Occupancy in excess of 100 percent means putting beds in corridors. It also means scheduling patients for major surgery without an available empty bed. The patient is prepared for surgery as an ambulatory patient, goes into the recovery room after surgery, and there waits for hospital bed assignment. If a bed does not open up by the time he needs to be moved, the administrative and nursing staff review the patient list to see who can be sent home, to another hospital, or to an extended care facility.

If the back-up schedule is too large, the staff reviews the elective surgery schedule and postpones operations that "will keep." Every postponement of this sort creates a public relations problem. The staff recognizes that the patient has cause to complain, the patient does complain, and he has the staff's sympathy. Making arrangements at home and work to go into the hospital is often as difficult for the patient as is finding a bed for the staff. In the eyes of union representatives who call or write Kaiser Health Plan representatives about such member grievances, there is only one source of error— bad management. Occasionally, Mr. Kaiser himself is blamed. But one nurse may have put her finger on a modern trend arising from the imbalance of demand and supply: "The patient has to give a little, too." On the other hand, interviews with directors of nursing gave little indication patients are well informed on what to expect.[16]

"The patient has to give a little, too." What a marvelously expressive phrase! How consoling it must be for those who daily witness the inconveniences and indignities—the long waits, the mixups over lost records, the hospital admissions requested but refused, etc.—that too many patients in pre-paid group practices have to put up with. Why don't advocates of Health Maintenance Organizations warn the American people that they, as patients, will have "to give a little, too"?

There is a similar spirit in physician staffing. Mr. Board-man writes that for each 100,000 members Kaiser-Permanente attempts to have thirty-four internists, ten general practitioners, fifteen pediatricians, ten obstetricians and gynecologists, eight general surgeons, three orthopedists, three neurosurgeons, one neurologist, two urologists, two dermatologists, one anesthesiologist, three radiologists, etc. This is possibly what the late Dr. Weinerman had in mind when he referred to the "Noah's ark" medical organizations "which assemble one or two varieties of every known species of medical specialist under one roof, regardless of the distribution of needs in the community." But statistical averages are useful only for large groups and over long periods of time. What happens in a Kaiser-Permanente group when, by chance, there is a sudden pileup of say, neurological illnesses requiring a neurologist? With one neurologist for 100,000 members the result is that the patients must wait their turn and such waiting may last weeks or even months. In 1970 Dr. Sidney Garfield told me that a Kaiser-Permanente patient might have to wait up to four months to see a particularly scarce specialist. So long as the patients served by a prepaid group conform to the statistical averages, all may be well. But when the patients defy the statistics they have to pay a high price in waiting time for their temerity. Of course when such a pileup occurs, a prepaid group may refer the excess patients to outside physicians and pay them on a fee for service basis. But that is an unanticipated financial drain, not likely to be undertaken lightly or often.

Good medical care involves more than economics. Ideally it should involve human rapport between patient and physician. Such rapport undoubtedly occurs in many patient-physician encounters in prepaid group practice but it can hardly be the rule. As Kaiser-Permanente and HIP operate, they are basically mass merchandisers of standardized medical care packages. They contract for thousands of patients at a time with local or state governments, with the federal government, with unions, and with employers. To the patients secured this way, the prepaid group practice has one overriding virtue, it costs little or nothing out of pocket for care. In return the patient accepts a very limited choice of physician and, often, impersonal treatment. It was all summed up for me by the mimeographed instructions I saw in one Kaiser-Permanente hospital in the Los Angeles area. Those instructions told patients how to make appointments: "Lift the telephone receiver and when the operator answers give her your number." There is no malice here, simply the fact that the efficiency experts long ago determined it is easier to keep track of human beings if they are identified by numbers rather than by names. The Internal Revenue Service also learned that lesson a long time ago.

It is true that many prepaid groups attempt to have patients get a family physician, a primary doctor to whom they will go first every time. But getting the physician one wants is frequently impracticable. A new patient may have been told by a friend that some Dr. Smith is a good doctor. When he enrolls the new patient may ask for Dr. Smith but at times he may be told Dr. Smith is booked up and is accepting no new patients. Even if the patient gets the Dr. Smith he wants, when he makes a later appointment for some reason he may find that to see Dr. Smith he will have to wait several weeks while if he is willing to see Dr. Jones —whom he has never seen before—he can get an appointment in a day or two or three. And Dr. Smith can hardly feel responsible for his patients in the way a private family doctor does. Dr. Smith is a hired employee or a partner who has agreed to work only a certain number of hours. One reason Dr. Smith may have joined prepaid group practice may be because he does not want to be bothered at night or on weekends or on vacations by his patients' problems. "Let whoever is on duty worry about them," is the slogan. It is all a bureaucratic atmosphere which attracts those who prefer a bureaucratic life with its fixed hours, limited responsibilities, and curtailed income. Some prepaid group doctors work overtime and try to establish personal relationships with patients. But they are all cogs in a large organization, and the bureaucratic atmosphere does not encourage such unusual effort.

Kaiser-Permanente officials understand the problem and worry about it. Here is the commendably candid statement by Dr. Herman Weiner, medical director of the Southern California Permanente Medical Group:

The responsibility of meeting the patient more than halfway—of understanding him as a person—is shared by all doctors. Some special manifestations of that need are peculiar to our organization. Historically, patients expect to pay doctors on a fee for service basis. When the health service is prepaid, the patient may have the feeling, during the immediate experience with his doctor, that he is not paying for treatment. The corollary, in the minds of many pa-

tients, is that what you don't pay for has little worth. Patients have
to be re-educated to the economics of our type of health care delivery.

Because of the size of our organization, we are extremely sensitive to the problem of depersonalization, and we try to do a number of things to offset it [He gives a number of examples such as
dispersing small hospitals throughout the area served] . . . In
every way possible—sometimes at the cost of maximum efficiency
—we try to create a climate in which the patient coming in for
medical care is known and knows that he is known.

I do not mean to present our strategy for meeting our responsibilities to the patient as though it were a mission accomplished. I
could wish that a great many things were different—that physicians' office hours were scaled to the patient's convenience more
realistically and that patients did not have to wait as long as they
sometimes do for appointments, particularly in some of our less
well staffed specialties. We have a long way to go, but we do recognize the presence of the challenge and we are geared to meet it.[17]

Dr. Weiner, a staunch advocate of prepaid group practice,
emphasized, "I do not think it is the only way or the inevitable way. It is not necessarily true that all group practice is,
by virtue of that condition, good, nor that physicians in
solo practice are necessarily failing their patients."

The real test of any medical arrangement is what happens in the patient-physician confrontation. Kaiser-Permanente, HIP and other prepaid group officials may worry
about personalizing care and making it high quality, but
what happens on the firing line? We have already referred to
the explosion of complaints at a meeting of HIP members
in the Washington Heights area in Manhattan. In an earlier
chapter we called attention to the extremely frequent prescription of aspirin substitutes and tranquilizers by Kaiser-
Permanente physicians in Northern California. One more
concrete example of what happens is available from a study
by two Kaiser-Permanente therapists, the chief psychologist

and the chief psychiatrist at the Kaiser-Permanente facilities in San Francisco. The study was designed to test means of referring patients for psychiatric help, but its findings are also illuminating on what happens in the patient-physician confrontation in this type of medical organization.

Briefly stated, the two researchers identified—through psychological tests and study of patient records—a group of 822 Kaiser-Permanente patients who probably needed psychiatric referral. The identification was made as part of a multiphasic screening physical examination whose results were to be turned over to internists who would discuss the findings and their significance with the patients involved. Just before the experiment began, all the internists concerned had the nature of the experiment explained to them. In particular they were told that half the patients involved would have notations suggesting psychiatric referral on their record and the other half—a control group—would not.

The results of the experiment were illuminating indeed. Six months after the initial examinations, of the 411 patients whose records contained an implied recommendation for psychiatric referral, only five had actually been seen by a psychiatrist. This was exactly the number of persons who had seen a psychiatrist from among the other 411 patients who had no such suggestion on their record. Moreover, only about half of the 411 patients for whom psychiatric referral was suggested had actually been referred by their internists. Ten—one-third—of the internists involved testified later they had never even noticed any notation on a patient record implying need of psychiatric consultation. Of the twenty internists who saw the suggestion on one or more of their patients' records, eight made no referrals, four referred all such patients, and eight referred half or more. The two experimenters' report on the internists' reactions seems worth pondering by anyone who thinks that the form—prepaid group practice—predetermines one high quality standard of medical care for all:

> Reasons given for reluctance to refer centered mostly about the physician's feelings regarding having to deal with an emotional problem when his time with the patient was limited. He felt he would open a "Pandora's box" that could not appropriately be handled in the fifteen minutes alloted for the initial return visit. . . . Ultimately, the internist's individual procedure regarding referral to psychiatry seemed little affected by the consider-rule [i.e., by the record notation implying need for psychiatric referral]. Physicians who routinely and easily refer to psychiatry continued to do so in the experiment, while physicians who usually do not refer to psychiatry essentially ignored the consider-rule. For the most part, it was the individual physician's mode of practice that mattered.[18]

It is all to the credit of those who direct Kaiser-Permanente that they authorized this experiment and permitted the publication of the results, for the findings are sobering indeed. There is explicitly admitted the fact that physicians in this system feel the pressure of limited time and avoid doing some things they might want to do if they had ample time. The suspicion must be strong that the ten internists —one-third of the total, remember—who missed seeing any note about psychiatric referral on their patients' records were delinquent because of the pressure of time. But what else did they miss under the pressure of the 15 minutes allotted for seeing the patient?

Then there is the final conclusion that what actually happens depends entirely upon the physician and his individual mode of practice! Yet those who see prepaid group practice and HMO as miracle instruments prate unceasingly about the ease of referral in these organizations and the high quality of care supposedly guaranteed by continual peer review. To quote the late Dr. Weinerman again: "Group conferences, medical audits, and informal office consultations are, in my experience, more common in the descriptive literature than in daily practice."

The emphasis on the negative in the preceding pages is not meant to damn the Kaiser-Permanente organization. Having talked to Kaiser-Permanente officials, doctors, and patients and having visited a number of their attractive hospital and office buildings, I am convinced that there are many virtues as well as problems in this remarkable organization. Moreover my personal experience has been that those I have contacted in Kaiser-Permanente have been willing to speak candidly and even to make available information not entirely to the organization's credit. The leaders of Kaiser-Permanente have made a major contribution with their remarkable achievement in privately organizing their extensive system, raising the necessary capital, and providing large amounts of perfectly acceptable care to their two million plus members. They have never claimed that they had the final and only perfect formula for solving the United States' problems in medical care. I know from private conversations that Kaiser-Permanente executives are embarrassed and appalled by the exaggerated claims made for prepaid group practice and the HMO concept. "Our members also die," was the way one Kaiser-Permanente executive put the matter in dismissing the fantasies of the enthusiasts. Kaiser-Permanente's requirement that members of groups being offered the chance to join that organization must also have offered to them at least one alternative health care plan is testimony to the realization that the Kaiser-Permanente mode of practicing medicine does not satisfy everybody and is not a universal formula.

Even more serious weaknesses exist in the Health Insurance Plan of Greater New York (HIP). It has organizational weaknesses Kaiser-Permanente has avoided, notably its heavy reliance (70 percent) upon physicians who work for HIP only part time and conduct their own private practices which, inevitably, some doctors must favor at the expense of HIP patients. Until very recently HIP did not own any hospitals; its patients were at the mercy of the gamble represented by the search of each HIP group's doctors to find a place to hospitalize their patients as hospitalization became necessary. Moreover there is evidence suggesting very unequal levels of care among different HIP medical groups.

Ironically, wide public realization of HIP's deficiencies did not take place until early 1972 and then only as a result of efforts by HIP's leadership to improve the quality of its care and eliminate some of the problems. To do this, HIP in 1971 negotiated with its independent medical groups to get two chief improvements: (1) regionalization, or merger of small medical groups into larger groups having better facilities and a larger selection of doctors and a more complete representation of different specialists, and (2) the conversion of all HIP physicians to a completely full time basis so as to eliminate the competition between a doctor's fee for service patients and his HIP patients who in general pay nothing beyond their basic subscription fee. To accomplish these and other desired improvements, HIP found it had to ask for a 36 percent increase in rate for members under sixty-five, i.e., other than Medicare patients. This increase was sought for 1972. A high HIP official has stated that an additional 30 percent rate increase was planned for 1973.

So long as HIP had seemed an inexpensive source of medical care, New York City officials—whose predecessors in the late 1940s had pressed for HIP's organization and whose employees and their families accounted for 300,000 of HIP's almost 750,000 members—did not concern themselves very much. In 1971, as a matter of fact, these officials sought to force many New York City employees to shift from Blue Shield to HIP and were deterred only by vigorous protests from city workers' unions. It turned out then that many of the workers liked their private physicians and did not want to change.

The 1972 HIP request for a 36 percent increase meant the city would have to pay HIP an additional $7 million for coverage of its employees in the plan. This ended official complacency; New York City's desperate financial situation put its officials in no mood to accept the increased cost. At a hearing called by the State Superintendent of Insurance to review the request for the 36 percent increase, New York City Personnel Director Harry I. Bronstein spoke of HIP as having "many already overcrowded and oversubscribed group centers" and he referred to "the long waits and crowded conditions" suffered by HIP members. His department had received a "substantial volume of subscriber complaints" and he declared that "an independent medical audit system (physicians, accountants, etc.) must be developed to evaluate past, present, and proposed future services." On HIP's proposal for expanding its experimental multiphasic screening program, he asserted, "This diagnostic unit has extremely high unit costs, and at this point it is by no means a closed case that the multiphasic approach has significantly greater benefits than more traditional diagnostic services." Recalling that at the time of HIP's 1969 rate increase there were promises of new and improved services, he said, "We would like to know which of those promises were kept and how many new and improved services were provided. Have we been paying for services we should have received and did not? Are we being asked to pay again for quality services we were supposed to get and didn't get?" He closed his statement with an implied threat that if the rate increase were approved, New York City might no longer offer HIP as an alternative health service available for the city's workers.[19]

The struggle over HIP's proposed reorganization also exposed another problem facing the HMO proponents. It became apparent that many HIP physicians were not enthusiastic about the planned changes. Officially, a spokesman for the recalcitrant doctors feared that the large rate increase would result in the loss of many HIP subscribers and make the organization less viable. The spokesman argued that the changes should be spread over a five year period so that the smaller but annual rate increases could be more readily absorbed. In conversation with me, he noted that another, more fundamental, fear moved many of his constituents. One of the changes HIP proposed was that it take over the physical premises and equipment at the various medical centers where HIP physicians practiced. The protesting doctors apparently believed this would change the balance of power between themselves and the HIP administrators, and be the first step on a road that could end with the physicians little more than hired employees subject to orders from nonphysician bureaucrats. HIP officials, on the other hand, argued that the protesting doctors really resented being compelled to go on a full time basis; that they preferred the combination of guaranteed minimum income represented by their part time commitment to HIP plus the opportunity to earn additional income by seeing private patients. To that point one HIP doctor replied that for years he and his colleagues had been subsidizing their work at

HIP by seeing private patients. Whatever the rights and wrongs of this particular dispute, it underlined the fact that those who would organize HMOs will face problems in recruiting physicians so long as private, fee for service practice is available as a viable alternative.

The State of New York Insurance Department's decision on the HIP rate increase request was released on May 25, 1972. It reflected full realization of the dilemmas posed before HIP and also before government officials who prefer prepaid group practice to conventional medical care. On the one hand, the Insurance Department granted HIP a rate increase averaging 29 percent, not too far below the 36 percent HIP had asked for. On the other hand, the Insurance Department raised the question of "whether the regionalization program will be the salvation of HIP or its demise," and said the answer "is unclear from the evidence." And as a sign of its concern about the situation, the Insurance Department imposed three specific requirements upon HIP. First, it required that HIP set up a special regionalization reserve account containing the portion of the rate increase allowed for this purpose. Second, it barred any expenditure from this reserve "until there has been a further submission to the Department with respect to the scope and timing of the [regionalization] program." Finally, the Department required that "prior to such submission, HIP conduct further discussion with its large customers (including the City of New York) with a view to ascertaining the extent of the willingness to pay for the costs of the regionalization program."

HIP's crisis was partially resolved in mid-August 1972. HIP agreed to accept only a 15 percent rate increase from New York City, though this obviously involved scrapping all earlier financial plans based on a higher rate increase.

HIP's president and executive vice president resigned, and remained silent as they were assailed publicly for having failed to clear HIP's expansion plans with its customers beforehand. Effective HIP leadership was taken over by a union leader, William Michelson, who denounced the excess fat in HIP's central administration and asserted his belief the organization's money woes could be solved by cutting $1.5 million from administrative expenses. He announced that the radical reform would be frozen for the time being, and HIP would continue using many part-time doctors for an indefinite period. He also revealed that HIP's perilous situation had resulted in turning for possible help to Blue Cross and Group Health Insurance Inc., both of which had made offers of aid and collaboration that could lay the foundation for possible future merger of HIP with one or the other organization.

One last point about the HIP experience is relevant here. The great bulk of the 36 percent increase HIP asked for was intended to improve the quality of service rather than to increase the quantity of services offered. This suggests that those who used HIP rates earlier as one basis of estimates for the costs of an HMO were misled because those earlier rates represented a level of services—in terms of quality—that HIP's own administrators regarded as unsatisfactory. This point is particularly important because much of the discussion of HMOs suggests that their advocates wish to take on broader, more inclusive and therefore more costly functions than present prepaid group practices offer. Hence we have visible two sources of possible understatement of HMO costs: (1) what might be called the quality differential required, as in the HIP case, to permit present prepaid group arrangements to give more satisfactory service and (2) the expansion factor, the cost of providing

still more ambitious coverage and care than have historically been offered by Kaiser-Permanente, HIP, etc.

The point may be made more explicit by considering
some of the requirements for an HMO in the bill sponsored
by Senator Kennedy in March 1972. Senator Kennedy
called for a thirty day open enrollment period each year
during which an HMO will have to accept individuals in
the order in which they enroll. He made the specific point
that this provision was intended to give individuals having
high health care needs access to HMOs. But present prepaid group practice organizations try to avoid enrolling
many individuals whose care is certain to be expensive and
cost more than the individual will pay in premium. They do
this either by restricting enrollment to groups or by requiring a medical examination for individuals wishing to enroll
separately, and rejecting those in bad health. Thus the possibility arises that under this scheme HMOs would be
loaded with people with cancer, heart disease, serious arthritis, and the like, while people in good health—who had
no reason to expect excessive medical bills—would prefer
to stay with private doctors working on a fee for service
basis.

Senator Kennedy made plain, too, his desire to bring
residents of poverty areas into the mainstream of medical
care by having them cared for in HMOs. But no HMO, he
argued, should have more than 50 percent of its membership from poverty areas. Yet almost all present experience
in prepaid group practice has been with working people
who are not only able to pay their way, but who have none
of the special medical and social pathology afflicting ghetto
dwellers. To treat the poor of the ghetto adequately will
cost more than it has cost until now to treat the average

union member belonging to Kaiser-Permanente or HIP.

Finally, it is an impressive and even awesome burden Senator Kennedy would place on HMOs. Here is his description of his proposal:

> The bill requires an HMO to deliver a comprehensive range of services. "Comprehensive health services" means a minimum range of services which must be offered by an HMO before it may qualify for assistance under this title. "Comprehensive health services" include health services provided without limitation as to time or cost as follows: "Physicians' services, inpatient and outpatient hospital services; extended care facilities services; home health services; diagnostic laboratory and diagnostic and therapeutic radiologic services; physical medicine and rehabilitative services—including physical therapy; preventive health and early disease detection services; emergency health services; reimbursement for expenses incurred for out-of-area health services when medically indicated; mental health services with an emphasis on the utilization of existing community mental health centers; dental services, with an emphasis on preventive dental health services for children; prescription drugs; and such other additional personal health services as the Secretary may determine are necessary including services dealing with alcoholism and drug abuse.[20]

Whatever one's view of Senator Kennedy's program, one thing should be clear: in these and other respects what he is urging is substantially more quantitatively, and therefore more expensive, than what present prepaid-group practices are providing. The expansion of services and the less selective population served, if the Kennedy proposal becomes law, will make a mockery of any cost estimates based on Kaiser-Permanente and HIP as presently constituted. The HMO, in short, could become a device for increasing national medical expenditures—both absolutely and as a percentage of national income—rather than for reducing those expenditures as so many HMO advocates argue.[21]

We can look back and see the nature of the HMO illusion. It is the belief that somehow the magic of a rigidly organized medical care system can produce better care, more care and, in total, cheaper care. The evidence simply does not justify that conclusion once it is realized that a national HMO system would have to include the seriously ill, the elderly, and the poor as well as selected elite populations like union memberships. The economies in one direction —reduction of hospital stays and of some questionable surgery—would be offset by the increased demand for medical care arising from prepayment and the increased administrative costs inherent in bureaucratic organizations.

What is most astounding about the push for HMOs is the insensitivity to the spirit of the times. We live in an age of alienation, when millions are suspicious of huge organizations which reduce them to numbers on punched cards. And nowhere are human contact and sympathy more important than in medicine where so many people want, above all, a "doctor who will listen." Yet unavoidably an HMO with thousands of patients, with doctors working on rigid appointment schedules so they can see their required quota of patients, must be an organization in which most patients are numbers and in which most doctors will seek to avoid the "Pandora's box" of a patient's unhappiness by prescribing Darvon Compound or Valium or Miltown. One has only to look at the alienation in American education to see the consequences of huge organizations malfunctioning and failing to meet the needs of those they serve. The call everywhere in America today is for decentralization, for breaking large units into small units, for reducing giant bureaucracies to human size so the individual can feel at home with them. But in medicine—where the individual doctor working on a fee for service basis does provide a decentralized, human-sized, non-punchcard directed service —the political pressure is all the other way toward repeating the errors of bureaucratic gigantism that have gotten us into the present mess in so many fields of American life.

The point is not that HMOs are evil or that those connected with them are either incompetent or unfeeling. It is rather that millions of Americans today enjoy better care —in terms of human contact, of genuinely knowing their doctor, of being listened to when they go for a consultation, of having choices—than they would have if forced to join an HMO. And similarly any forced collectivization of doctors, any economic or other compulsion to force physicians to give up private practice and become cogs in large HMO machines would stir up enormous resentment that could not help but be reflected in millions of patient-physician meetings.

By all means organize HMOs. By all means let us have competition and multiple choices for consumers needing or desiring medical care. But let it be fair competition, not a race in which one form of medical care is heavily subsidized and favored by government while another is taxed and harried and disparaged in a thousand ways. For some patients and some physicians, the HMOs are undoubtedly adequate and satisfactory; for others they will be systems of torture and grave dissatisfaction. In so delicate, complex, and little understood an area as the emotional and physical health of human beings we cannot afford to be dogmatic and arrogant. We need to go slowly; to experiment in a wide variety of situations; to leave as wide an area of choice as possible. But will the politicians—men enamored of simplistic slogans and inaccurate clichés—understand that it is much easier to ruin what is now in many respects the world's best medical system than to improve it? As this is written the question is still open but watching Senator Kennedy or like-minded politicians in action on this matter gives reason for discouragement. The myth that government can produce magic answers dies hard, despite debacle after debacle in education, housing, mail service, military production, and other areas. Must American medicine become another disaster area before the lesson is learned?

NOTES

1. E. Richard Weinerman, "Problems and Perspectives of Group Practice," in Ray H. Elling, editor, *National Health Care*. Chicago/New York: Aldine Atherton, 1971, pp. 212–13.
2. Anne R. Somers, editor, *The Kaiser-Permanente Medical Care Program*. New York: The Commonwealth Fund, 1971, p. vi.
3. *Medical World News,* October 29, 1971, p. 39.
4. Marjorie Smith Mueller, "Independent Health Insurance Plans in 1970," Research and Statistics Note, U.S. Department of Health Education, and Welfare, Social Security Administration, Office of Research and Statistics, March 22, 1972.
5. Nora Piore, Deborah Lewis, and Jeannie Seeliger, *A Statistical Profile of Hospital Outpatient Services in the United States: Present Scope and Potential Role*. New York: Association for the Aid of Crippled Children, August 1971 (mimeographed).
6. Department of Health, Education, and Welfare, *Towards a Comprehensive Health Policy for the 1970's A White Paper*. Washington: May 1971, p. 33.
7. Somers, *op. cit.,* p. 4.
8. *Ibid.,* p. 117.
9. *Ibid.,* p. 21.
10. Greer Williams, *Kaiser-Permanente Health Plan Why It Works*. Oakland, California: The Henry J. Kaiser Foundation, February 1971, p. 52.
11. Somers, *op. cit.,* p. 38.
12. Williams, *op. cit.,* p. 38.
13. John M. Glasgow, "Prepaid Group Practice as a National Health Policy: Problems and Perspectives," *Inquiry,* March 1972, pp. 8–11.
14. John J. Boardman, Jr., "Utilization Data and the Planning Process," Somers, *op. cit.,* p. 69.
15. *Ibid.,* p. 65.
16. Williams, *op. cit.,* pp. 25–26.
17. Somers, *op. cit.,* pp. 93–94.
18. Nicholas A. Cummings and William T. Follette, "Psychiatric Services and Medical Utilization in a Prepaid Health Plan Setting: Part II," *Medical Care,* January–February 1968, p. 36.

19. *Statement by Harry I. Bronstein, City Personnel Director and Chairman, City Civil Service Commission on the HIP Rate Increase Request,* April 24, 1972 (mimeographed).
20. *Congressional Record,* March 13, 1972, p. S 3780.
21. On this point see also Glasgow, *op. cit.,* pp. 11–12.

CHAPTER VII

LESSONS FROM ABROAD

Many critics of American medicine mount a two-front attack. They not only assail what they consider the serious weaknesses of this country's medical care organization, but they point to one or more foreign countries as offering a more perfect model that should be emulated here. Thus one New York newspaper columnist argued in 1971 that the United States should adopt the British system of socialized medicine. We have referred earlier to the admiration for Soviet medicine expressed by Robert G. Kaiser, *Washington Post* Moscow correspondent. The very title of the CBS television documentary, "Don't Get Sick in America," might suggest to some that it was good to get sick anywhere else. One critic buttresses his admiration for the British by telling of an American visitor who had serious surgery and spent weeks in a British hospital and paid nothing for it. Another critic tells us of an American victim of kidney disease who returned to his native Sweden because he could get the renal dialysis he needed free of charge.

The harsh truth is that nobody knows how to design an ideal medical system, one that simultaneously is inexpensive, combats all possible ailments effectively, quickly separates the genuinely ill from the malingerers and is considerate of the time and convenience of patients, doctors, and nurses. All medical care is part necessity and part luxury but there is no universal agreement, nor is there ever likely to be, as to where the line should be drawn. Our ignorance was well stated by a team of American, British, and Swedish medical economists who, in the mid–1960s, carefully studied the three national medical systems and came to this modest, agnostic conclusion:

There is considerable evidence that our choices on priorities for provision of medical care are not made on a well-informed basis. Furthermore, with the wide differences which exist, all three countries cannot have reached correct conclusions unless the medical needs of our populations vary to a highly improbable degree. If lower utilisation rates suffice to deal with morbidity in one country, then others may be wasting resources. On the other hand it is also possible that greater provision results in reduced disability.

Present information does not suffice to permit a judgment as to whether we are prodigal with our resources, or whether our provisions for care are appropriate or even insufficient.[1]

What can be demonstrated is that in countries with radically different medical systems from that in the United States, there is a good deal of dissatisfaction with socialized medicine and a yearning for some of the benefits of private, fee for medical service that are so often scorned and ridiculed in the United States. We have already quoted Alexander Solzhenitsyn to that effect in his comments on the Soviet medical system in *Cancer Ward,* so let us turn to Britain and Sweden.

In Britain, shortly after World War II, the National Health Service was created as a system of socialized medicine divided into two parts. One provides ambulatory care through access to family physicians who treat minor illnesses. The second part consists of hospital care during which the patient is cared for by specialists, cut off entirely from his family physician. All this is "free," i.e., paid for through the tax system. Nevertheless, private medicine persists in Britain and there are about 2 million subscribers to various insurance schemes that pay for private medical services.

One major reason for the growth of private medical practice in Britain, where all must pay taxes to support the National Health Service, is simply the long waiting lines for admission to hospital for nonemergency conditions. In early 1972 the National Health Service had a list of about 500,000 people waiting for what was officially called noncritical surgery but which probably seemed more important than that to the people affected.[2] When they pay for their care directly, British citizens can choose when they will go into the hospital and get operated on more quickly than if they wait for the National Health Service waiting list to reach their name—a matter often of one or two years. They can pick their own surgeon, rather than accept being operated on by whichever surgeon, resident, or intern is available when their turn comes up. Naturally the opportunity for those with means or private medical insurance to jump the queue inspires resentment and produces proposals from time to time that private practice be abolished. But the fact that leading Labor Party as well as Conservative politicians use private practitioners provides important support for Britain's private medical practice. Here is the recent judgment of the London Times on this subject:

The National Health Service has been in existence now for nearly a quarter of a century, but private practice continues and seems likely to remain a permanent part of the British medical scene. So it should. To suppose that all patients ever can be treated absolutely equally in every respect is an illusion. It would be manifestly absurd for a Cabinet Minister not to be able to have a minor operation at the time of his choice. Some priorities are bound to be determined on non-medical grounds. . . . The practical question is not whether there should be a private medical sector, but how large it should be.

Because the health service is so under-financed there is a strong case for encouraging the growth of private medicine. . . .

The reference to the underfinancing of the British National Health Service reflects a chronic complaint in countries with socialized medicine. Once medicine has to be paid for through the national budget, it has to compete for funds with all the other demands on a government's resources. The medical service's claims for money and other resources have to be weighed against national defense, education, the environment, the police forces, etc., etc. In Britain, as we noted earlier, one resolution of the problem for many years was the decision not to build any more hospitals, though the population was increasing and though numerous technical advances in medicine made the therapeutic possibilities of hospital care ever greater. Major political battles have been fought from time to time over proposals for easing the financial strain on the national budget by having patients pay part or all of the cost for such items as drugs and eyeglasses.

It is interesting that the British chose to build their structure of primary physician care on a system of individual general practitioners, rather than on a group practice model similar to that of Kaiser-Permanente. From time to time complaints are heard that at least some of these British general practitioners are overburdened, give only superficial care and are so removed from the mainstream of general medicine that they are of little use to their patients. Thus the medical advisor of a major British company wrote recently that "people do approach directly doctors in private and industrial practice because the patient perceives his own doctor as having no time and/or interest in the patient's concern that he is and remains fit." [4]

The operation of the British National Health Service has clearly failed to attain one much-desired result: It has by no means eradicated differences in length of life or infant mortality based on socioeconomic differences. Even in the socialized British medical system the upper and middle classes live longer and their infant children die less frequently than the poorest groups in the population. In England and Wales in 1930–1932, i.e., before medicine was socialized, mortality among males fifteen to sixty-four— taking mortality for all of them as one hundred—varied only from an index of 90 for the top socioeconomic class to an index of 111 for the lowest social class. But in 1959 –1963 the mortality ranged from an index of 76 in the top group to 143 in the lowest. The United Kingdom Registrar General's analysis complained, "The most disturbing feature of the present results when compared with earlier analyses is the apparent deterioration in social class V [the lowest social class] . . . whilst the mortality of all men fell at all ages except seventy to seventy-four, that for social class V men rose at all ages except twenty-five to thirty-four." The British Government was so displeased by the variation in infant mortality found among social classes in 1959–1963 that it sought to hide the facts by lumping together the data for the two highest and the two lowest social classes. Nevertheless even with this expedient it turned out that infant mortality in the two lowest social classes was almost 50 percent higher than in the two highest social classes.[5] Those who believe that somehow or other it is all the fault of private, fee for service medicine in

the United States that the poor in this country have lower
longevity and higher infant mortality than more fortunate
economic groups might ponder this evidence that such
major differences persist even in a twenty-five year old socialized medical system in as relatively wealthy and advanced a country as Britain.

Finally, British socialized medicine has had no more
luck in stemming the overall rising death rate from degenerative diseases than the private doctors of the United
States. Here are the statistics for the seven chief causes of
death in Great Britain, the data being standardized mortality ratios with 1950–1952 = 100, i.e., the period used for
comparison is the early years of the operation of the National Health Service: [6]

	Men		Women	
	(1950–1952 = 100)			
Cause of Death	*1961*	*1967*	*1961*	*1967*
Arteriosclerotic heart disease	141	158	144	160
Central nervous system vascular lesions	99	92	96	89
Pneumonia	125	118	134	138
Cancer of lung, bronchus and trachea	157	180	138	183
Bronchitis	105	91	66	47
Cancer of stomach	87	79	78	66
Cancer of breast	minor		102	106

In April 1972 I visited Stockholm to try to get some first
hand information about the Swedish medical system. I
knew that Sweden had for many years enjoyed one of the
world's lowest infant mortality rates, while Swedes of both
sexes have traditionally had one of the highest life expectancies in the world. I knew also that American physicians

often spoke highly of the training and competence of their Swedish colleagues. Finally I had seen many invidious comparisons made in American publications between the "free" medicine of Sweden and the "expensive" medicine of the United States.

I received a cordial welcome from Bengt Janzon, director of information for the National Board of Health and Welfare which sets overall policy for the Swedish medical system. Mr. Janzon soon made plain that he was pained by any notion that the experience of a small, homogeneous nation like Sweden was directly applicable to much larger and more heterogeneous countries. To illustrate his point, he told this story: Some years ago a group of Swedish physicians visited India and were told about one of that country's health problems. Eager to help, the Swedes told their hosts how Sweden handled the matter. The Indians then asked the Swedes how many people their country had. Informed that Sweden had 8 million people, the Indians replied that that number was about the right size for a small laboratory experiment in India.

Mr. Janzon explained that the Swedish medical system is almost fully nationalized. Only 1,300 of the country's 11,-000 doctors remain in private practice. They are still very busy and still do very well financially. Most medical care in Sweden is now centered about government-owned hospitals which dispense both inpatient and outpatient care. For an outpatient visit, a Swede pays less than $1.50 and his maximum payment for drugs prescribed by a doctor on any one visit cannot exceed about $3. Hospital care is provided without direct payment. But Mr. Janzon made no attempt to hide the fact that the entire system was expensive and was paid for through substantial payroll and sales taxes. He was proud of the system but conceded it had at least two problems: a shortage of doctors, which he hoped would end by 1975, and a tendency of physicians to prescribe too many tranquilizers, a tendency the government was seeking to combat. Mr. Janzon indicated he thought physicians in the Swedish socialized medical system were paid very well, particularly top administrators who receive the same salary as the Prime Minister, 150,000 crowns annually. He also reported that the cost of the Swedish medical system had been rising very rapidly in recent years.

A friend of mine in Sweden suggested that if I wanted to know what the ordinary Swede thought of his medical system, I should read the articles on the subject in the Stockholm newspaper *Expressen* which had run a lengthy exposé March 5–9, 1972. I got those issues and found the articles a collection of horror stories centering about these themes: the incredible difficulty of getting into a hospital, the long waits for hospitalization and the suffering and injury caused sick people by the shortage of hospital beds. If *Expressen* is to be believed, Sweden also has a "health care crisis" and the articles were as one-sided in emphasizing the negative as are typical American journalistic attacks on the United States "health care crisis."

When I spoke to individuals resident in Sweden—Swedes and Americans—I found the disenchantment expressed in the newspaper reflected also in the comments of these informants. Even Stockholm's taxicab drivers seemed to have few kind words for their country's socialized medicine. I could not believe my ears when one informant, in response to my question, said: "Don't get sick in Sweden. You have never seen such impersonal care and such long waits in your life. Every time you go to the clinic, you see a different doctor. And if you're hospitalized and are seen by a physician three times in one day, it will almost certainly be three different doctors." I was told of a foreign ambassador who was refused hospitalization even though he had a heart attack, of a veteran Swedish diplomat whose child lost the use of a thumb because of a long wait for care in a clinic to which the child's distraught mother had brought him after an accident. Another informant told me, "If you want to get into a hospital, tell them you're hemorrhaging. That usually works." In short, I discovered that socialized medicine in Sweden had overloaded the medical system precisely as had socialized medicine in Britain and the Soviet Union. The results were waits of up to two years for nonemergency operations, long waits in clinics and refusal to hospitalize even very sick patients whose required care was medical rather than surgical.

The Swedish doctors I spoke to complained of the bureaucracy they had to contend with and of the flood of patients clamoring for clinic service and hospital admission. Here is the way one of Sweden's most eminent physicians —a ranking administrator in Stockholm's socialized medical service—described what happened in his country after reforms introduced on January 1, 1970 substantially increased the dominance of socialized medicine:

All hospital physicians were deprived of their right to see private patients in consultation; with the exception of professors, they all got working hour schedules of about fifty hours a week in the hospitals. By means of other legislation, their security on the job is lessened, and the avenue to political appointments instead of appointments based on evaluation of training and competence is being opened. . . .

This new system does not offer substantial incentives for doctors to do a superior job. There are, no doubt, a few physicians who feel that the absence of "economic transactions" between them and their clients make life easier, but I believe that in the majority of cases the doctor-patient relationship has become weaker in a situation where the patient is no longer seeing the doctor of his or her choice, but an impersonal institution, in which one cannot be assured of meeting one's "own" doctor. My feeling is that incentives are being reduced in a socialized system, and unless you introduce incentives other than economic, you are going to get a service that is worse, and not better, than what we used to have.

A reflection of this situation is the fact that waiting lists have been substantially increased during 1970 for admission to hospital outpatient departments and so useless for admission to certain clinical departments (such as departments of medicine) that they are almost not in use. Two-thirds to three-fourths of all admissions to departments of medicine take place as emergencies, in many instances emergencies among those who were on the waiting list. Waiting time in our outpatient department has doubled in 1971, and this is true also of other departments. One of the reasons for this is precisely that "socializing" of physicians in ambulant care makes them less interested in the work-up of the more difficult patients, who are, instead, increasingly being referred to hospitals. It is, of course, equally true of the Swedish system as it is of the American that patients will be seen by a doctor "at any time," inasmuch as this refers to emergency units in hospitals. Otherwise, it is, of course, not true. Doctors in both countries are increasingly unwilling to work outside office hours or to make house calls. This is a consequence of the present trends in the affluent society at large, where—as taxes rise—leisure becomes a more and more valued commodity.[7]

Some, no doubt, will want to dismiss the testimony of the author, Dr. Gunnar Biorck, as simply the bitter complaint of a physician denied the right to practice privately. But since Dr. Biorck, an internationally renowned physician, is a key figure in Swedish medicine and could enter private practice if he wished, this seems too cynical a verdict. All I can testify is that the Swedes I spoke to—a small sample, true, but covering a variety of economic groups— seemed far from happy with their socialized system and

with the taxes they had to pay for the entire welfare society
in their country.

Then why does Sweden rank so very high in world international health comparisons? Persons I interviewed in
Stockholm made the following points: Sweden is a small,
prosperous, homogeneous society with none of the depths
of poverty found in American ghettos. The harsh Scandi-
navian climate over the centuries has tended to produce a
present population with excellent genetic qualities from the
point of view of health and longevity. The Swedes, I was
told, have a passion for exercise and for the outdoor life
which contrast sharply with the life styles of millions of sedentary Americans. The Swedish Government has one of
the world's severest laws—and enforcement mechanisms
—against drunken driving. When people are going to a party
where they expect to drink alcohol, I was told, they come
and go by cab or by public transport and leave their cars
home. They know that they run the risk, if they drive, of
being stopped at random by the police who will test their
breath to see if they have been drinking recently, and those
discovered driving with only a small quantity of alcohol in
their blood will be punished by severe jail terms or large
fines and suspension of their driver's licenses.

Britain and Sweden, in short, have not created medical
utopias by socializing their medical care systems. Both societies carry heavy tax burdens for the "free" care they dispense. In both societies, the queues of persons waiting for
hospital admission are long, far longer than Americans
would find acceptable. In both countries those who can do
so prefer to go to private practitioners for the personal care
that does not flourish in an impersonal socialized system.
Many Americans—though obviously not all—get better,

more convenient, and more personalized care than is available to the great majority of Britons and Swedes, and those Americans would find either the British or the Swedish system represented a deterioration in the quality of their medical care. Many of those Americans, one may suspect, would not be consoled by the knowledge that they were paying for medical care through heavier taxes, rather than through direct payment to the physician they chose.

NOTES

1. Osler L. Peterson *et al.*, "What Is Value for Money in Medical Care? Experiences in England and Wales, Sweden, and the U.S.A.," *The Lancet,* April 8, 1967, p. 776.
2. *The Times* (London), April 27, 1972.
3. *Ibid.,* March 30, 1972.
4. Letter of Joseph L. Kearns in *The Lancet,* January 22, 1972, p. 209.
5. Julian Tudor Hart, "Data on Occupational Mortality, 1959–1963, Too Little and Too Late," *Ibid.,* p. 192.
6. Central Statistical Office, *Social Trends* Number 1, 1970. London: Her Majesty's Stationery Office, 1970, p. 109.
7. Gunnar Biorck, "An Insider's View of Medicine in Sweden," *Modern Medicine,* August 9, 1971, p. 45.

CHAPTER VIII

POLICIES FOR
THE FUTURE

Among many American physicians today there is an attitude of resentment and pessimism about the future. As one doctor put it, "We can't win. Whatever we do, it's wrong in the public mind. We're damned if we do, and we're damned if we don't." The case of Harold E. Wagner helps explain this widespread bitterness.[1]

Mr. Wagner, a fifty-four-year-old machinist from Elida, Ohio, was a patient awaiting an eye operation in Detroit's Harper Hospital the morning of December 1, 1971 when he developed signs of heart failure. First his heart beat became wildly erratic and a specially trained emergency team of eight physicians and nurses and technicians worked successfully for two hours to shock his heart back to normal rhythm with a machine called a defibrillator. Then, aware that he had had an earlier heart attack and was still in grave danger, his doctors sought to assess the damage to Mr. Wagner's heart by putting him through a complex X-ray procedure called coronary arteriography. This disclosed a complete obstruction of the right coronary artery and a three-quarters obstruction of the left coronary artery; the blood vessels carrying essential nutrients to the heart were almost closed off. To try to save Mr. Wagner, it was decided to construct shunts around the obstructed areas so as to provide new blood channels to the heart. To perform this procedure—which is less than a decade old—the surgeons transplanted arteries from Mr. Wagner's leg to his chest. After five hours—it was now almost 10 P.M. that same eventful day—the operation was finished and Mr. Wagner was still alive, the blood supply to his heart vastly improved. But then his heart beat returned to its earlier erratic pattern and at 10:07 P.M. that night he died.

During the last twelve hours of Mr. Wagner's life he was attended by fifteen physicians, including, among others, a general internist, two cardiac surgeons, a cardiologist, a pathologist, a radiologist, a neurologist and an anesthesiologist, as well as by numerous nurses and technicians. He received thirty-one units of blood that day, i.e., his blood supply was replaced almost four times in the frantic battle to save his life. Yet he died.

From one point of view, this is a stirring and impressive story. An ordinary worker—Mr. Wagner's salary was $7,700 a year when he died—had had every resource of modern science marshalled to help him. In all probability neither the President of the United States nor a multimillionaire could have received much better care from more highly trained people than Mr. Wagner did in his desperate situation. For him, in his last hours, there was no shortage of doctors, of nurses, of modern equipment, of blood or of any other essentials medical care could provide. He died, but it was not because of lack of expert, devoted effort.

It was from another point of view, however, that the case was presented to the American people. Testifying before a Senate subcommittee investigating health insurance, Leonard Woodcock, president of the United Automobile Workers, called the cost "scandalous." The bill came to $7,311 and after Mr. Wagner's hospital insurance, blood donations by his friends, and waiver of fees by some of the physicians involved, Mrs. Wagner was left with a bill of more than $1,-000 she could not pay. The headline writer pronounced his judgment: "Modern Medical Price: Death and Bankruptcy for One Man's Family." Clearly, what the doctors involved at the time had seen as a heroic effort to save a fellow human being's life had been transmuted into another count in the general indictment against the American medical system.

Were the doctors at fault for making the effort to save Mr. Wagner? After all, they could have decided that he was too far gone and that there was no point in attempting heroic measures to rescue his heart. If they had, would Mr. Woodcock have been testifying before some Congressional committee about the "heartless doctors" who would not use the latest achievements of science for an ordinary worker? Was the hospital at fault for having available the expensive, modern equipment needed to make the attempt? If that equipment had not been available, might Mr. Woodcock have called the lack of this equipment "scandalous"? As the doctor quoted above put it, "We're damned if we do, and we're damned if we don't."

For Mr. Woodcock the answer to such tragedies as that of Mr. Wagner is national health insurance. But we have seen earlier that to make medical care "free" is to flood the medical system and permit the "worried well," as Dr. Garfield has termed them, to usurp resources needed by the sick. It is interesting to speculate whether such extreme efforts to save Mr. Wagner would have been made if he were in a hospital run by a prepaid group. Death, we noted earlier, is the ultimate economy.

There is, of course, a milder and more feasible solution to such financial problems as those that arose in the Wagner case. A national system of catastrophic illness insurance—perhaps the type advocated by Senator Russell Long or along the lines suggested by Professor Martin Feldstein in the material quoted earlier—would have avoided the problems faced by Mr. Wagner's widow. It would seem an obvious solution in this case and in many of the other tragic situations propagandized by advocates of national health insurance. Yet, curiously, catastrophic insurance has been hotly attacked by both the left and right extremists in the medical spectrum. On the left, catastrophic insurance is opposed since it would take much of the steam out of the left's drive to alter radically the American medical system and perhaps ultimately socialize it. On the right, there is the fear that once a catastrophic insurance law took effect, it would provide an entering wedge which some succeeding Congress would finally turn into "free" medical care for all. Yet it has much to commend it to anyone who looks at the problems faced by the very sick.

Like everything else, catastrophic insurance would solve some problems but also bring some other problems with it. It is not unreasonable to fear that catastrophic insurance would further skew American medicine in the direction of the most complex and most expensive types of care. Moreover, it might have the potentials for encouraging the survival—at great cost and with no hope of restoration to health—of many extremely ill persons whose bodily functions had been taken over by respirators and other modern supportive equipment. In short catastrophic insurance would have to be accompanied by a mechanism for making decisions as to when enough was enough, for example, when some comatose vegetable that had once been a vi-

brant human being should be permitted to die. No one need
envy the individuals charged with making such decisions
but they can be made and are, in fact, made every day by
physicians and relatives. In any case, I believe that passage
of catastrophic illness insurance legislation with appropriate
safeguards and limitations would repair a key weakness of
American medical insurance.

We turn now to the central issue in the national debate on
medical policy to which this study seeks to contribute. This
is the call for comprehensive national health insurance—
"free" medicine for all—and a radical restructuring of the
American medical system so as to eliminate the private
practice of medicine by individuals or small groups and replace them by "medical systems" of the Health Maintenance Organization type. National health insurance could
be passed without restructuring the delivery of care, but the
chief political thrust comes from those who aim at both
objectives. For those who want these twin objectives, it is a
positive gain if national health insurance alone is adopted
and results in chaos because the existing medical system is
overloaded. In 1933 many German Communists welcomed
Adolf Hitler's ascent to power, reasoning that his reign
would be brief and they would succeed him. So, today, reason many enemies of what they call the "medical nonsystem." Professor David Mechanic has written of those "who
desire radical changes in the structure of health services,
and who see no politically viable approach to obtaining
such modifications at the present time" and who therefore
"believe that the conditions for such change can develop by
overloading the health services system to such a degree that
a public clamor develops for a radical restructuring of the
entire health field." [2] In short there are those who, primar-

ily for ideological reasons, want to collectivize America's hospitals and physicians and who don't mind seeing medical chaos in this country if that is necessary to achieve their goal. They have apparently learned nothing from the disaster Russia suffered for more than thirty years between Stalin's collectivization of the Soviet peasant in the early 1930s and the period in the late 1960s when Soviet collectivized agriculture finally began to work with a minimum reasonable modicum of efficiency and productivity.

The most widely discussed proposal for national health insurance, and the project which has received the ardent support of labor unions and forces to the left of the unions, is the bill introduced by Senator Kennedy in the Senate and by Representative Martha Griffiths in the House. The Kennedy-Griffiths bill would go a long way toward socializing American medicine by creating a system of compulsory national health insurance financed entirely by federal taxes. It would seek to encourage prepaid group practice at the expense of traditional fee for service. It would also seek to control costs by a system of regional health budgets with which this country has no experience. Enactment of this bill would be the most radical change in the long history of American medicine. This writer's distaste for that proposal has been made plain earlier. It may be useful, therefore, to present here the evaluation of more sympathetic observers, the authors of the Brookings Institution's recent valuable study, *Setting National Priorities: The 1973 Budget*. The Brookings authors believe the Kennedy-Griffiths plan "has many advantages. It would establish one system of medical care for all—with all the social and economic advantages of a single system." I would argue that a single medical care system for all would have very great disadvantages as well, but that disagreement is not major at this point. More important is the sober evaluation of the problems of the Kennedy-Griffiths proposal which the Brookings study presents immediately after lauding that legislation. It seems worthwhile to reproduce this analysis of the consequences of "free medical care for all" in full:

But the Kennedy-Griffiths program also raises problems. Because it would provide free medical care not only to the poor but to all of the population, it would move into the federal budget a huge component of private outlays for normal medical expenses that are now being made by middle- and upper-income groups with no major financial strain. Financing this would require large tax increases that would be devoted not toward accomplishing objectives attainable only in the public sector, but toward substituting public outlays for private outlays that would have been undertaken in any event. If the large tax increases necessary to finance the program were adopted, it is highly unlikely that additional taxes could be raised to meet the costs of other high priority public objectives.

Other difficulties would arise from the abandonment of private payments for most medical services and the introduction of complex regulatory mechanisms to control the prices and uses of services. There are more than 7,000 hospitals in the United States, more than 20,000 nursing homes and several hundred thousand physicians. The kinds of practice, costs, types of services, and quality of care vary greatly from area to area and within each area. The establishment by administrative bodies of equitable and appropriate fees would be a task of Herculean proportions, particularly on a nationwide scale. Controlling costs would also require the control and monitoring of services rendered. Utilization review committees would have to be established to determine whether stays in institutions were unnecessarily long. Similarly, it would have to be determined whether physicians were ordering unnecessary tests as a means of increasing their incomes, requesting unnecessary repeat visits, referring patients unnecessarily to additional physicians, and so on. At present the technical capability for monitoring the entire health care system is simply not available. [And it would be very expensive, if available, as well as introducing many undesirable frictions. HS]

Some of the controls proposed in the Kennedy-Griffiths bill are novel and imaginative—the concept of a fixed budget to be allocated among regions, and new methods of encouraging the capitation and HMO approach to financing and delivering medical care. But they are as yet untested. Experimenting with those approaches in existing federal health insurance programs in selected areas might yield valuable information. However, to carry them out all at once in a nationwide system of medical care could pose *major risks*. [Italics supplied. HS]

The last major concern with the Kennedy-Griffiths plan is the impact it would have on the health care services provided to low-income people. Unlike other plans that specifically subsidize the care of the poor and the near poor, this plan would give everyone equal financial access to medical care—that is, care would be free for all. But this alone would not guarantee that everyone would have equal access to care. Instead, at least initially, the plan might widen the disparity among income classes in the use of medical services. A changeover to free care would represent a greater reduction in the price of care to higher-income persons. Many of the poor currently receive free care or reduced cost care through Medicaid or charity. The largest increases in demand therefore might come from higher-income groups. Moreover, medical manpower and facilities are much more abundant in higher-income areas. Unless deliberate steps were taken to increase the supply of these resources in low-income areas, the poor would have less physical access to care. While these problems might be overcome in time, the result of providing free care to all might paradoxically be to increase care most for those who can already afford it.[3]

Professor Theodore R. Marmor of the University of Wisconsin has made an important and more general related point in his 1971 testimony before the House Ways and Means Committee:

Were I asked the question, "Which of the major national health insurance bills do you favor?" I would answer, "None of them."

. . . such exaggerated claims have been made on all sides that one does not have the basis for a sober estimate of the suggested programs; $70 billion programs are compared with $10 billion ones, all on one convenient page. Pressure groups present convenient manageable summaries of schemes which would allegedly change the face of American medicine. Cost estimates are thrown around as if they were seeds at spring plowing. And claims are made about the desirable consequences of private health insurance, HMOs, national capitation schemes, and so forth which are difficult to accept on the basis of the evidence that advocates present. My simple conclusion is that we don't yet know enough to choose the appropriate means of government health insurance.[4]

The point is essential because the American medical care system with its four million workers, its more than 200 million patients and potential patients, its incredible array of specialized skills and equipment, and its billions of dollars of capital investment is quite simply the most complicated industry in the United States. To suppose that we know enough to improve it through radical changes imposed upon this system in a brief period is fantasy more appropriate to an LSD "trip" than to sober legislative deliberation. There must be a high probability that radical changes imposed quickly and in a manner that disregards the interests of key groups could create chaos and seriously worsen the average quality of American medical care.

One would suppose that legislators would have learned from the unsatisfactory results of so many recent past disappointments. This past decade the United States has seen many humanitarian efforts initiated to improve social conditions, efforts generously financed through government budgets, yet efforts that failed. The "war against poverty" did not end poverty. Numerous "innovative" programs to improve the education of ghetto children turned out to have shockingly little success in improving the reading, writing, and arithmetic of the intended beneficiaries. Medicare and Medicaid produced little change in the nation's mortality statistics but contributed powerfully to the inflation of medical costs. Very expensive housing programs to help the poor often turned out mainly to enrich the speculators and finance the corruption of government housing inspectors. It is no wonder that many liberals who had started out with such high hopes for the possibilities of quick reform and improvement have had second thoughts. There has developed what Dr. Alice M. Rivlin, a former HEW Assistant Secretary for Planning and Evaluation, has called "a new realism about the capacity of a central government to manage social action programs effectively." Dr. Rivlin has described the evolution of her thinking in these terms:

I, for one, once thought that the effectiveness of a program like Headstart or Title I of the Elementary and Secondary Education Act could be increased by tighter management from Washington. Something was known about "good practices," or effective ways of reaching poor children; more could be learned and transmitted to the local level through federal guidelines and regulations and technical assistance. As knowledge accumulated the guidelines could be tightened up, and programs would become more effective.

This view now seems to me naive and unrealistic. The country is too big and too diverse, and social action is too complicated. There are over 25,000 school districts, and their needs, problems, and capacities differ drastically. Universal rules are likely to do more harm than good. Nor, given the numbers of people involved, is it possible simply to rely on the judgment or discretion of federal representatives in the field.[5]

The implications of this sobering experience for the nation's medical care system are immediate. The medical care system is even more complicated than the school system; different localities are at least as diverse in their medical resources and needs as they are in their educational "needs, problems, and capacities." The same caution Dr. Rivlin indicates she has learned about quick educational reform directed from Washington would seem to be justified regarding hopes for quick medical reforms directed from Washington.

The key point here has been made by Dr. Charles L. Schultze of the Brookings Institution who was formerly President Johnson's Director of the Budget:

> A national medical program cannot at one and the same time guarantee virtually all the medical care private citizens can demand regardless of income, provide a financial mechanism and a set of incentives that hold down escalation of costs, and avoid comprehensive detailed regulation of medical care by Washington bureaucrats.[6]

Put another way, Dr. Schultze is saying that a national system of "free" medical care would require many universal rules set down in Washington, and Dr. Rivlin has already told us, "Universal rules are likely to do more harm than good." The prospect must be faced that if any of the comprehensive schemes for radically changing the American medical system becomes law, the result could be disastrous. In the face of this prospect is it unreasonable to ask even the most ardent reformer to make haste slowly, to experiment carefully before imposing radical changes upon this great and diverse nation, and to ponder the many advantages of evolutionary change as compared to revolutionary change?

We have argued above that the American medical system is much better than is usually assumed, and we have warned against radical Khrushchev-like sudden changes in this very complex mechanism. But none of this implies that American medicine is perfect, that the status quo must be preserved intact, or that improvement is impossible. Our plea here, rather, is for intelligent change applied where change is needed and will improve matters, for "patching up" and remedying the weaknesses of a basically sound mechanism, and for change at a pace that will permit the numerous interests involved—providers and consumers alike—to compromise their differences and work out mutually tolerable, if not always mutually ideal, compromises.

Reasonable critics of the American medical system have centered their fire on two problems: (1) The high and rapidly increasing cost of medical care and (2) the difficulties of access to this care in some areas and for some population groups.

On the first issue a historic change has taken place since mid-1971. The imposition of wage and price controls has nowhere produced so dramatic a result as in medicine. Formerly the medical care component of the Consumer Price Index was the most inflationary element in the cost of living. This past year the rise in this component has been cut more than half, and the rise has actually been less than the overall increase in the CPI. No doubt a sudden lifting of all wage and price controls would produce a sudden upward surge in all fields, including medical care. But such an abrupt return to the free market seems unlikely while underlying inflationary forces are still strong. It has now been proved that the growth of medical care prices can be curbed effectively as part of a national comprehensive control program aimed at slowing inflation. The lesson will not be easily forgotten, though it remains to be seen how long individual health care providers will be willing to accept the highly discriminatory controls now in effect. Nor can it be ignored that an increasing number of hospitals are complaining that controls now in effect threaten them with bankruptcy. Thus it is certain that there will be problems ahead, but it may be doubted that the runaway behavior of hospital costs which followed the introduction of Medicare and Medicaid will be allowed again. As for doctors' fees, the rapid increase in the number of physicians entering practice in this country should provide useful assistance for those concerned with restraining price increases for medical services. Unless, of course, Congress substantially extends the scope of "free" medical care paid for through the tax system.

But, of course, certain types of medical care are inherently expensive. No one can give first-class and up-to-date treatment of a serious heart attack, kidney failure, lung cancer, disabling stroke or the like cheaply. The real costs involved must be great for any medical system, costs in terms of skilled manpower and of modern equipment needed to help each patient maximally. Only a system of catastrophic medical insurance—designed, perhaps, along the lines Professor Feldstein has suggested —can meet the inevitable financial problems in this field. But even here, as we have noted earlier, there must be limits to prevent expensive abuses.

On the issue of improving access to medical care, a number of approaches are available. Certainly the shortage of physicians and other health care personnel in America's "inner cities" and in many rural areas must be alleviated, while more financial support is needed for the hospitals and other medical facilities serving these deprived areas. Some increase in the network of OEO Neighborhood Health Centers would seem to be useful. But quicker results might be obtained by providing greater resources for the Public Health Service's National Health Service Corps which now is providing physicians and other health care personnel for more than 100 communities in the nation.[7] Other approaches also need to be explored. Tax incentives might be offered physicians and other health care personnel deciding to practice in certain designated shortage areas. The medical profession might think of creating a new tradition of national service that would obligate every physician to serve for some specified period—say at least three months every decade —in some domestic area of special need. Certainly the numerous American physician volunteers who have served the civilian population in Vietnam and who have worked on the medical ship *Hope* have set precedents that should be useful in helping to meet the most urgent domestic needs.

More generally, there is almost unanimous agreement that there exists serious geographic and specialty maldistribution of the nation's physicians. The medical profession has an obligation to move more energetically on this front. A drastic reduction of training programs in specialties already afflicted with a sharp oversupply of personnel would be one step. Another would be action to increase the status of primary physicians and to increase their number. Service for several years as a primary physician might be made a requirement for specialty training. Financial aid might be offered to physicians in specialties that are overmanned so as to encourage these physicians to retrain in family medicine or other deficit specialties. And the medical profession might designate certain geographic areas that are best supplied with physicians as "areas of doctor surplus" and attempt to discourage other physicians from moving into the surplus areas for some periods of time.

Of course there are other specific areas of American medicine that need improvement. The gross inadequacies of the nation's system of emergency medical aid must be corrected by providing more personnel, more facilities, and more transport vehicles so that better and quicker care can be given to victims of automobile accidents, heart attacks, strokes, and the like. In many of these situations, timely intervention of skilled care can make the difference between full recovery and death or very serious, permanent disability.

The present scandalous situation in the provision of blood for transfusions must be radically improved. Today, because of the unwillingness of most Americans to contribute blood, hospitals and physicians must depend to an alarming degree upon commercially bought blood which often carries with it an unacceptably high risk of transmitting hepatitis, malaria, and other diseases. By a major effort of popular persuasion and the introduction of new incentives—probably including an income tax credit for blood donations—this country must seek to have all blood for transfusions provided voluntarily so as to minimize the risks borne by those who receive this blood.

One additional development deserves mention here: The American Medical Association is encouraging the development of peer review organizations at the local level, organizations designed to protect the public and the government against physicians who are either incompetent or venal. Coincidentally, there is increasing formal pressure on doctors to continue their self-education while engaged in practice. In the United States, there are multitudinous opportunities for physicians to keep current with the latest developments in their fields of interest. The means for self-education range from reading the vast numbers of medical periodicals and new medical books constantly being published, through attendance at professional meetings where the latest developments are stressed, to enrollment in special short courses held throughout the country to update the knowledge of those who attend. Many physicians have always availed themselves of these opportunities. Now the laggards are coming under increasing fire from their colleagues to do the same.

As discussed earlier, excessive hospitalization and unnecessary surgery have been matters of increasing public concern in recent years. Such efforts as the Certified Hospital Admission Program (CHAP) in California's Sacramento County and the Hospital Admission and Surveillance Program (HASP) in Illinois are illustrative of techniques aimed at checking such abuses, techniques which are spreading throughout the United States, especially in areas where medical care foundations are operating. Particularly useful in this activity are the data on hospitalization and surgery collected and disseminated by the Professional Activity Study (PAS) of the Commission on Professional and Hospital Activities in Ann Arbor, Michigan.

Outside the delivery system, there are at least two other priority areas: (1) The nation's financially shaky medical education system must be put upon a firmer basis and restructured so that it can do far more than it does now to assure the continuing lifetime professional education of practicing physicians and to create a medical career ladder in which able and industrious people can move upward in medical responsibility and economic rewards. (2) The deterioration in the nation's medical research mechanism—the wonder and envy of the rest of the world—must be reversed since improved future medical care is possible only if we know much more about preventing and curing the main present scourges of mankind than we do now.

But it is not to changes in the medical system that we must look for the quickest results in improving the nation's health over the next decade. The most important road to better health and greater longevity for Americans lies in fundamental changes of lifestyle away from patterns that conduce to sickness and early death and toward new patterns that promote well being. Cutting air pollution, changing the American diet to cut down consumption of cholesterol-rich foods, alcohol, and drugs, effective gun control, new and more responsible attitudes toward driving and the provision of safer automobiles—these measures can be far more effective than a thousand HMOs in improving the health and well being of Americans. For the poorest Americans, what is required is alleviation of their poverty in ways that promote their integration as useful members of society. So long as people are plagued by poor nutrition, poor housing, inability to compete for useful jobs, and the other despair-producing conditions of their lives, their fundamental ills will be beyond anything the most skilled physicians can permanently cure.

If the reader had hoped to find here simple, easy answers for a medical utopia, he will be disappointed. There are no utopias in real life and the improvements we make are soon devalued by rising expectations and new demands. Yet the American medical system—pluralistic, complex, and ever-changing—has served the American people well. It can continue to do so if the aim of change is to increase the choices of both health care providers and those who need their help. Those who would collectivize American medicine to satisfy their ideological preferences would have cause to regret the result when they themselves required medical care for serious illness.

NOTES

1. *New York Times,* May 21, 1972.
2. David Mechanic, "Problems in the Future Organization of Medical Practice," *Law and Contemporary Problems,* Spring 1970, p. 234.
3. Charles L. Schultze, Edward R. Fried, Alice M. Rivlin and Nancy H. Teeters, *Setting National Priorities: The 1973 Budget.* Washington, D.C.: The Brookings Institution, 1972, pp. 248–50.
4. *National Health Insurance Proposals.* Hearings before the Committee on Ways and Means, House of Representatives, 92nd Congress First Session on the subject of National Health Proposals. Washington: U.S. Government Printing Office, 1972, part 4, pp. 826–27.
5. Alice M. Rivlin, *Systematic Thinking for Social Action.* Washington, D.C.: The Brookings Institution, 1971, pp. 123–24.
6. *Saturday Review,* January 22, 1972.
7. Ralph M. Thurlow, "A Bright New Hope for Doctor-Short Areas," *Medical Economics,* May 8, 1972, pp. 234–35. *New York Times,* May 24, 1972.

SELECTED BIBLIOGRAPHY

Odin W. Anderson, *The Uneasy Equilibrium* (New Haven: College & University Press, 1968).

Carnegie Commission on Higher Education, *Higher Education and the Nation's Health* (New York: McGraw-Hill, 1970).

Raymond S. Duff and August B. Hollingshead, *Sickness and Society* (New York: Harper & Row, 1968).

Marvin H. Edwards, *Hazardous to Your Health* (New Rochelle, N.Y.: Arlington House, 1972).

Rashi Fein, *The Doctor Shortage An Economic Diagnosis* (Washington, D.C.: Brookings Institution, 1967).

Martin S. Feldstein, *The Rising Cost of Hospital Care* (Washington, D.C.: Information Resources Press, 1971).

Eliot Freidson and Judith Lorber, eds., *Medical Men and Their Work* (Chicago/New York: Aldine-Atherton, 1972).

Eli Ginzberg with Miriam Ostow, *Men, Money & Medicine* (New York: Columbia University Press, 1969).

Edward M. Kennedy, *In Critical Condition: The Crisis in America's Health Care* (New York: Simon and Schuster, 1972).

Herbert E. Klarman, *Medical Economics: Essays and Articles* (The University of Iowa: Graduate Program in Hospital and Health Administration, 1969).

Herbert E. Klarman, *The Economics of Health* (New York: Columbia University Press, 1965).

John H. Knowles, ed., *Hospitals, Doctors, and the Public Interest* (Cambridge: Harvard University Press, 1965).

Robert J. Myers, *Medicare* (Homewood, Ill.: Richard D. Irwin, 1970).

Mark V. Pauly, *Medical Care at Public Expense* (New York: Praeger Publishers, 1971).

Alice M. Rivlin, *Systematic Thinking for Social Action* (Washington, D.C.: Brookings Institution, 1971).

William R. Rosengren and Mark Lefton, *Hospitals and Patients* (New York: Atherton Press, 1969).

William R. Roy, *The Proposed Health Maintenance Organization Act of 1972* (Washington, D.C.: Science and Health Communication Group, 1972).

Charles L. Schultze, Edward R. Fried, Alice M. Rivlin, and Nancy H. Teeter, *Setting National Priorities: The 1973 Budget* (Washington, D.C.: Brookings Institution, 1972).

Anne R. Somers, *Health Care in Transition: Directions for the Future* (Chicago: Hospital Research and Educational Trust, 1971).

Herman M. Somers and Anne R. Somers, *Doctors, Patients and Health Insurance* (Washington, D.C.: Brookings Institution, 1961).

Anne R. Somers, ed., *The Kaiser-Permanente Medical Care Program: A Symposium* (New York: The Commonwealth Fund, 1971).

Rosemary Stevens, *American Medicine and the Public Interest* (New Haven: Yale University Press, 1971).

Greer Williams, *Kaiser-Permanente Health Plan: Why It Works* (Oakland, Cal.: Henry J. Kaiser Foundation, 1971).

INDEX